THE NA~~~
KECK FUTURES INITIATIVE

SMART PROSTHETICS

EXPLORING ASSISTIVE DEVICES FOR THE BODY AND MIND

TASK GROUP SUMMARIES

Conference
Arnold and Mabel Beckman Center of the National Academies
Irvine, California
November 9-11, 2006

THE NATIONAL ACADEMIES PRESS
Washington, D.C.
www.nap.edu

THE NATIONAL ACADEMIES PRESS   500 Fifth Street, N.W.   Washington, DC 20001

NOTICE: The task group summaries in this publication are based on task group dis-cussions during the National Academies Keck *Futures Initiative* Smart Prosthetics: Ex-ploring Assistive Devices for the Body and Mind Conference held at the Arnold and Mabel Beckman Center of the National Academies in Irvine, California, November 9-11, 2006. The discussions in these groups were summarized by the authors and re-viewed by the members of each task group. Any opinions, findings, conclusions, or recommendations expressed in this publication are those of the task groups and do not necessarily reflect the view of the organizations or agencies that provided support for this project. For more information on the National Academies Keck *Futures Initiative* visit www.keckfutures.org.

Funding for the activity that led to this publication was provided by the W. M. Keck Foundation. Based in Los Angeles, the W. M. Keck Foundation was established in 1954 by the late W. M. Keck, founder of the Superior Oil Company. The Foundation's grant making is focused primarily on pioneering efforts in the areas of medical research, sci-ence, and engineering. The Foundation also maintains a Southern California Grant Program that provides support in the areas of civic and community services with a special emphasis on children. For more information visit www.wmkeck.org.

International Standard Book Number-13:   978-0-309-10466-1
International Standard Book Number-10:   0-309-10466-1

Additional copies of this report are available from the National Academies Press, 500 Fifth Street, N.W., Lockbox 285, Washington, DC 20055; (800) 624-6242 or (202) 334-3313 (in the Washington metropolitan area); Internet, www.nap.edu.

THE NATIONAL ACADEMIES
Advisers to the Nation on Science, Engineering, and Medicine

The **National Academy of Sciences** is a private, nonprofit, self-perpetuating society of distinguished scholars engaged in scientific and engineering research, dedicated to the furtherance of science and technology and to their use for the general welfare. Upon the authority of the charter granted to it by the Congress in 1863, the Academy has a mandate that requires it to advise the federal government on scientific and technical matters. Dr. Ralph J. Cicerone is president of the National Academy of Sciences.

The **National Academy of Engineering** was established in 1964, under the charter of the National Academy of Sciences, as a parallel organization of outstanding engineers. It is autonomous in its administration and in the selection of its members, sharing with the National Academy of Sciences the responsibility for advising the federal government. The National Academy of Engineering also sponsors engineering programs aimed at meeting national needs, encourages education and research, and recognizes the superior achievements of engineers. Dr. Wm. A. Wulf is president of the National Academy of Engineering.

The **Institute of Medicine** was established in 1970 by the National Academy of Sciences to secure the services of eminent members of appropriate professions in the examination of policy matters pertaining to the health of the public. The Institute acts under the responsibility given to the National Academy of Sciences by its congressional charter to be an adviser to the federal government and, upon its own initiative, to identify issues of medical care, research, and education. Dr. Harvey V. Fineberg is president of the Institute of Medicine.

The **National Research Council** was organized by the National Academy of Sciences in 1916 to associate the broad community of science and technology with the Academy's purposes of furthering knowledge and advising the federal government. Functioning in accordance with general policies determined by the Academy, the Council has become the principal operating agency of both the National Academy of Sciences and the National Academy of Engineering in providing services to the government, the public, and the scientific and engineering communities. The Council is administered jointly by both Academies and the Institute of Medicine. Dr. Ralph J. Cicerone and Dr. Wm. A. Wulf are chair and vice chair, respectively, of the National Research Council.

www.national-academies.org

THE NATIONAL ACADEMIES KECK *FUTURES INITIATIVE* SMART PROSTHETICS STEERING COMMITTEE

P. HUNTER PECKHAM (Chair)* (NAE), Donnell Institute Professor of Biomedical Engineering, Case Western Reserve University, and Director, FES Center, Veterans Affairs Medical Center

FRED H. GAGE (NAS/IOM),** Vi and John Adler Professor, Laboratory of Genetics LOG-G, The Salk Institute for Biological Studies

STEPHEN C. JACOBSEN (NAE/IOM),** Distinguished Professor of Mechanical Engineering, University of Utah

CATO T. LAURENCIN, M.D., Ph.D. (IOM),** University Professor, Lillian T. Pratt Distinguished Professor and Chairman, Department of Orthopedic Surgery, Professor of Biomedical Engineering, Professor of Chemical Engineering, University of Virginia Health System

MICHAEL M. MERZENICH (NAS),** Francis Sooy Professor of Otolaryngology, Keck Center for Integrative Neurosciences, University of California, San Francisco, School of Medicine

---

* Also Chair, Planning Committee.
** Also Member, Planning Committee.

THE NATIONAL ACADEMIES KECK *FUTURES INITIATIVE*
SMART PROSTHETICS PLANNING COMMITTEE

MARK ABEL, M.D., Professor of Orthopedic Surgery and Pediatrics, Director, Motor Analysis and Motor Performance Laboratory, University of Virginia

TREENA LIVINGSTON ARINZEH, Assistant Professor, Department of Biomedical Engineering, New Jersey Institute of Technology

SANGEETA BHATIA, M.D., Ph.D., Director, Laboratory for Multiscale Regenerative Technologies, Associate Professor, Health Sciences and Technology, Massachusetts Institute of Technology, Brigham and Women's Hospital

GYORGY BUZSAKI, M.D., Ph.D., Board of Governors Professor, Center for Molecular and Behavioral Neuroscience, Rutgers University

APOSTOLOS GEORGOPOULOS M.D., Ph.D. (IOM), Regents Professor, McKnight Presidential Chair in Cognitive Neuroscience, Director, Center for Cognitive Sciences, American Legion Brain Sciences Chair, Professor of Neuroscience, Neurology, and Psychiatry, University of Minnesota Medical School, Director, Brain Sciences Center, Director, The Domenici Research Center for Mental Illness, Veterans Affairs Medical Center

STEVEN GOLDSTEIN (NAE), Henry Ruppenthal Professor of Orthopaedic Surgery and Bioengineering, Associate Chair for Research, University of Michigan

WARREN M. GRILL, Associate Professor of Biomedical Engineering and Surgery, Duke University

SCOTT MAKEIG, Director, Swartz Center for Computational Neuroscience, University of California, San Diego

MRIGANKA SUR, Sherman Fairchild Professor of Neuroscience, Head, Department of Brain and Cognitive Sciences, Massachusetts Institute of Technology

Staff

KENNETH R. FULTON, Executive Director
MARTY PERREAULT, Program Director
MEGAN ATKINSON, Senior Program Specialist
ANNE HEBERGER, Research Associate
RACHEL LESINSKI, Senior Program Specialist

The National Academies
Keck *Futures Initiative*

The National Academies Keck *Futures Initiative* was launched in 2003 to stimulate new modes of scientific inquiry and break down the conceptual and institutional barriers to interdisciplinary research. The National Academies and the W. M. Keck Foundation believe that considerable scientific progress will be achieved by providing a counterbalance to the tendency to isolate research within academic fields. The *Futures Initiative* is designed to enable scientists from different disciplines to focus on new questions, upon which they can base entirely new research, and to encourage and reward outstanding communication between scientists as well as between the scientific enterprise and the public.

The *Futures Initiative* includes three main components:

Futures *Conferences*

The *Futures* Conferences bring together some of the nation's best and brightest researchers from academic, industrial, and government laboratories to explore and discover interdisciplinary connections in important areas of cutting-edge research. Each year, some 100 outstanding researchers are invited to discuss ideas related to a single cross-disciplinary theme. Participants gain not only a wider perspective but also, in many instances, new insights and techniques that might be applied in their own work. Additional pre- or postconference meetings build on each theme to foster further communication of ideas.

Selection of each year's theme is based on assessments of where the intersection of science, engineering, and medical research has the greatest potential to spark discovery. The first conference explored *Signals, Decisions, and Meaning in Biology, Chemistry, Physics, and Engineering.* The 2004 conference focused on *Designing Nanostructures at the Interface between Biomedical and Physical Systems.* The theme of the 2005 conference was *The Genomic Revolution: Implications for Treatment and Control of Infectious Disease.* In 2006 the conference focused on *Smart Prosthetics: Exploring Assistive Devices for the Body and Mind.* In 2007 the conference will explore *Aging and Longevity.*

Futures *Grants*

The *Futures* Grants provide seed funding to *Futures* Conference participants, on a competitive basis, to enable them to pursue important new ideas and connections stimulated by the conferences. These grants fill a critical missing link between bold new ideas and major federal funding programs, which do not currently offer seed grants in new areas that are considered risky or exotic. These grants enable researchers to start developing a line of inquiry by supporting the recruitment of students and postdoctoral fellows, the purchase of equipment, and the acquisition of preliminary data—which in turn can position the researchers to compete for larger awards from other public and private sources.

National Academies Communication Awards

The Communication Awards are designed to recognize, promote, and encourage effective communication of science, engineering, medicine, and interdisciplinary work within and beyond the scientific community. Each year the *Futures Initiative* honors and rewards individuals with three $20,000 prizes, presented to individuals who have advanced the public's understanding and appreciation of science, engineering, and/or medicine. Awards are given in three categories: book author; newspaper, magazine, or online journalist; and TV/radio correspondent or producer. The winners are honored during the *Futures* Conference.

Facilitating Interdisciplinary Research Study

During the first 18 months of the Keck *Futures Initiative*, the Academies undertook a study on facilitating interdisciplinary research. The study examined the current scope of interdisciplinary efforts and provided recommendations as to how such research can be facilitated by funding organizations and academic institutions. *Facilitating Interdisciplinary Research* (2005) is available from the National Academies Press (www.nap.edu) in print and free PDF versions.

About the National Academies

The National Academies comprise the National Academy of Sciences, the National Academy of Engineering, the Institute of Medicine, and the National Research Council, which perform an unparalleled public service by bringing together experts in all areas of science and technology, who serve as volunteers to address critical national issues and offer unbiased advice to the federal government and the public. For more information, visit www.national-academies.org.

About the W. M. Keck Foundation

Based in Los Angeles, the W. M. Keck Foundation was established in 1954 by the late W. M. Keck, founder of the Superior Oil Company. The Foundation's grant making is focused primarily on pioneering efforts in the areas of medical research, science, and engineering. The Foundation also maintains a Southern California Grant Program that provides support in the areas of civic and community services with a special emphasis on children. For more information visit www.wmkeck.org.

The National Academies Keck *Futures Initiative*
5251 California Avenue – Suite 230
Irvine, CA 92617
949-387-5783 (Phone)
949-387-0500 (Fax)
www.keckfutures.org

Preface

At the National Academies Keck *Futures Initiative* Smart Prosthetics: Exploring Assistive Devices for the Body and Mind Conference, participants were divided into interdisciplinary working groups. The groups spent eight hours over three days exploring diverse challenges at the interface between science, engineering, and medicine. The composition of the groups were intentionally diverse, to encourage the generation of new approaches by combining a range of different types of contributions. The groups included researchers from science, engineering, and medicine, as well as representatives from private and public funding agencies, universities, businesses, journals, and the science media. Researchers represented a wide range of experience—from postdoc to those well established in their careers—from a variety of disciplines that included orthopedic surgery, mechanical science and engineering, physical medicine and rehabilitation, biology, materials science, biomedical engineering, electrical engineering, chemistry, neuroscience, pharmacology, anatomy, robotics, genetics, and physics.

The groups needed to address the challenge of communicating and working together from a diversity of expertise and perspectives as they attempted to solve a complicated, interdisciplinary problem in a relatively short time. Each group decided on its own structure and approach to tackle the problem. Some groups decided to refine or redefine their problems based on their experience.

Each group presented two brief reports to the whole conference: (1) an interim report on Friday to debrief on how things were going, along with any special requests (such as an expert in neural stimulation); and (2) a final briefing on Saturday, when each group:

- Provided a concise statement of the problem;
- Outlined a structure for its solution;
- Identified the most important gaps in science and technology and recommended research areas needed to attack the problem; and
- Indicated the benefits to society if the problem could be solved.

Each task group included a graduate student in a university science writing program. Based on the group interaction and the final briefings, the students wrote the following summaries, which were reviewed by the group members. These summaries describe the problem and outline the approach taken, including what research needs to be done to understand the fundamental science behind the challenge, the proposed plan for engineering the application, the reasoning that went into it, and the benefits to society of the problem solution.

Contents

APPENDIXES

To view the preconference tutorial webcasts or conference presentations, please visit our website at www.keckfutures.org/prosthetics.

Conference Summary

Haley Poland, Graduate Student
Annenberg School of Journalism, University of Southern California

Whether they are helping a blind person see, a deaf person hear, or a double amputee walk, prostheses have come a long way since Captain Hook. What were once wooden limbs and glass eyes are now engineered electromechanical devices interfacing with human body systems and communicating, almost intelligently, with the human nerves and brain. For thousands of people living with disabilities, "smart" prosthetics could mean faster rehabilitation, more effective therapy, and even return to an independent life. From joint replacements, cochlear devices, and brain implants to artificial valves, hearts, and limbs, advancements in prosthetic devices are beginning to blur the line between technology and biology.

From November 9 to 11, 2006, more than 150 researchers in fields ranging from biomedical and material engineering to surgery, neurology, and military medicine converged upon the Arnold and Mabel Beckman Center in Irvine, California. The fourth annual conference of the National Academies Keck *Futures Initiative* (NAKFI), "Smart Prosthetics: Exploring Assistive Devices for the Body and Mind," challenged participants to determine just what "smart" means and how best to achieve that smartness in the future.

LEVELING THE FIELD

As smart prostheses are engineered structures designed to exist beside or within human physiology, the field is inherently interdisciplinary. The novelty of an interdisciplinary conference breeds enthusiasm, excitement, and innovative thinking, but such a conference also requires a common level of understanding on a wide range of topics. As Hunter Peckham, chair of the NAKFI Smart Prosthetics Committee aptly stated, "We've grown up in scientific silos." To bridge the gaps 13 overview tutorials presented the basics of the associated fields and the state of those fields in science today. For the first time since the NAKFI conferences began four years ago, the overview tutorials, intentionally broad to give the scientists familiarity with topics outside of their own expertise, were webcast live prior to the conference.

In one tutorial Robert Kirsch, associate professor of biomedical engineering at Case Western Reserve University, described and discussed systems for maintaining homeostasis—a balanced internal environment. He noted that a smart prosthesis should play the same homeostatic role in the body as whatever body part it's replacing. Simply stated, motor controls go out from the brain to the device as sensory feedback comes in—a closed loop.

Warren Grill, associate professor of biomedical engineering, neurobiology, and surgery at Duke University, walked conference participants through the basics of neural stimulation, which feeds information into the nervous system, and neural recording, which interrogates the nervous system to determine the internal state and could also provide command signals to a prosthetic device. In discussing how to improve orthotics to help people walk, Bradford Bennett, research director of the Motion Analysis and Motor Performance Laboratory and assistant professor of research at the University of Virginia, promoted patient-specific models that record and adapt to a person's individual gait.

Addressing a less technological but integral aspect of prosthesis development, Mark Humayan, professor of ophthalmology at the Keck School of Medicine, and Frances Richmond, director of the Regulatory Science program at the University of Southern California, outlined the rigorous regulatory process a medical device must go through on its path from benchtop to bedside. As Richmond emphasized, it's important to think about these processes as materials, components, and clinical trial methods are chosen during development. "If we choose the wrong path," she said, "we greatly delay and make more expensive our ability to get to a commercial market."

Two particularly captivating talks given were not overview tutorials but rather personal accounts from researchers who are also users of smart prosthetic devices. Alexander Rabchevsky, assistant professor of physiology at the Spinal Cord and Brain Injury Research Center at the University of Kentucky, lost use of his lower body due to a spinal cord injury in a motorcycle accident in the 1980s. In recounting his own trials with the surgically implanted functional electrical stimulation (FES) for standing, exercise, and transfers, Rabchevsky gave unparalleled insight into the life-changing impact prosthetic devices can have. After almost two decades lying down or in a wheelchair, the FES allows him to stand, if only for a few moments, and look his wife in the eye. Hugh Herr, associate professor of media arts and sciences at Massachusetts Institute of Technology, lost both legs below the knee to frostbite in a climbing accident when he was 17. A "better rock-climber with his specialized prostheses than he was before the accident," Herr now builds cutting-edge limb devices that use technology to harness and even improve upon the abilities of the human body. For both Rabchevsky and Herr their firsthand knowledge of prosthesis use contributes immensely to their research—as it did to the NAKFI conference.

Whenever everyone gathered in the auditorium over the course of three days, the unique temperament of the conference emerged. Often, a witty and well-timed joke made the audience erupt in rollicking laughter. At other times, during discussion of provocative or controversial topics, the auditorium resembled British Parliament or the trading floor of the New York Stock Exchange. But whether the group was in agreement or dissent, the variety of perspectives and the passion behind them were undeniable.

A MEETING OF THE MINDS

While the plenary tutorials and a question-and-answer panel provided a foundation from which to build, the 11 task groups were where the heavy lifting occurred. Over the course of the conference each intentionally diverse group was given eight hours to address a challenge question or statement. With the deadline fast approaching, groups contemplated plans to restore sensory perception of limb movement, design a prosthesis to grow with a child, replace damaged brain tissue, and design a functional tissue prosthesis. Others tackled problems like electrode longevity, the best way for electrodes to interface with the brain, and how hybrid prostheses might exploit electrical processes within nerve cells.

The level of expertise in each group meant highly technical discussions, and during the first two-hour session, more than a few people were looking at each other as if to say, "How is this ever going to come together?" In some rooms the groups were suspended by an uncomfortable tension as participants hesitantly hashed out where the discussion was headed and just who was going to head it. In other rooms effective collaboration created a synergy that had some enlivened scientists rocking in their chairs, like children who can't sit still. Remarkably, at the end of eight hours every group had a plan.

On the last day, during more than four hours of task group "report-outs" in the auditorium, a spokesperson for each group outlined the plan of attack. While some had developed preliminary models of material devices or structures, others had generated elaborate analyses of the most pressing science and technology gaps related to the group's challenge question. One group, asked to design a functional tissue prosthesis, diagrammed a renewable internal power supply for a prosthetic device. The hybrid-technology "battery pack" aimed to harness cellular energy by aligning electrocytes, coaxed to behave in a certain way, on an implantable, biocompatible platform. In troubleshooting the topic of brain electrodes, a group proposed tissue engineered, self-inserting bioelectrodes (which use neurons to interface with neurons), as well as optically based interfaces that make use of the photovoltaic properties of photosynthetic membranes. Another group asked, "Can brain control guide or refine limb control?" and started off their final presentation with a definitive answer: "Yes." What followed was a research plan to develop a device that could identify, capture, and decode neural signals when a patient intends to move a limb that is not really there.

In reality, the task groups were not expected to solve the complex quandaries placed before them. The group sessions served to catalyze interactions between fields by allowing a diverse group of people to pursue novel patterns of thought, free of the logistical delays of actual research. It's in this collaborative stumbling toward big ideas—in that faltering sense of direction—that the truly great strides take place. And, figuratively, that may mean going from Chicago to New York via Los Angeles. The value is in what was happened upon and who was met along the way.

The days were long, and conference goers, some admittedly drained of their day's supply of scientific inspiration, happily relaxed and networked during the receptions and dinners. It was during these periods that an invaluable outcome of the conference became evident: Relationships formed across disciplines. "I definitely met people that I'll be talking to very soon," said one scientist on the last day. "The important stuff happens after the conference."

For this reason the *Futures Initiative* offers an incentive for collaboration as part of its mission to promote innovative scientific investigation. Each year $1 million in seed grants, up to $75,000 each, are awarded competitively to conference participants wishing to pursue interdisciplinary research, learn new skills, or perhaps keep alive a fledgling dialogue begun at the conference. This year's grants will be announced in April 2007.

COMMUNICATING SCIENCE

While promoting interdisciplinary research sits at the top of the initiative's priority list, not far below is effective communication of scientific ideas and advancements to the general public. To make science understandable for a wide audience, science journalists usually find themselves whittling daunting and dizzying topic areas into digestible bites of accessible language. Making scientific complexity simple takes concerted time, effort, and practice. What better opportunity to hone such a skill than at an interdisciplinary conference on a subject like smart prosthetics? Accordingly, NAKFI invited graduate science writing students from universities across the country to attend the conference. Each science writer participated in a task group, and then wrote an article documenting the group's conclusions. The task group summaries are collected here to provide an overview of this integral part of the conference.

To further underscore the significance of effectively communicating science, the National Academies presented three $20,000 communications awards during dinner at the Beckman Center on November 9th. The communications awards acknowledge excellence in reporting and communicating science, engineering, and medicine to the general public. In the book category author Charles C. Mann received an award for *1491: New Revelations of the Americas Before Columbus*, a debunking of popularly held notions of the pre-Columbian Americas. Elizabeth Kolbert of *The New Yorker* was acknowledged for her three-part series *The Climate of Man*, on the science and politics of global climate change. Last, director Nic Young, producer Anna Thompson, and executive producer Bill Locke received a 2006 Communication Award for the History Channel and Lion Television's *Ape to Man*, a documentary overview of human evolution.

INTELLIGENT DESIGN

In the keynote address Michael Merzenich of the Keck Center for Integrative Neurosciences said, "We can make smarter prostheses when we're smarter in integrating state-of-the-art neuroscience with state-of-the-art engineering, medical, and social science." As was acknowledged during the conference, researchers cannot underestimate the capacity of the human brain—to restore function, to be trained, to make up for what's been lost in extraordinary ways. If with the help of prosthetic devices sensory information can continue to flow into the brain from the peripheral nervous system, research shows that the brain will learn to use that information for motor control. Now isn't it remarkable what a person (and a person's brain) can do with a little help?

Describe a Framework for Replacing Damaged Cortical Tissue and Fostering Circuit Integration to Restore Neurological Function

TASK GROUP DESCRIPTION

Background

With worldwide demographics increasingly shifting toward an aging population, neurological diseases are increasingly common. Stroke, for example, is now the third largest medical cause of death in the Western world, and among those who survive its ravages, nearly two-thirds become disabled. Furthermore, the effects of these disorders are particularly debilitating, due to their profound impact on sensation, cognition, and other tasks that are often central to the afflicted person's identity. To rise to this challenge an original therapeutic framework is needed to restore critical functions associated with damaged areas of the brain, either through the introduction of new tissue or other material into those areas or via the facilitated adoption of the original functions by new brain areas.

A promising target for such treatments is the cerebral cortex. In addition to vitally underpinning much of perception, movement, and executive function, the cortex has the additional benefit of retaining significant plasticity for change throughout the lifespan. Furthermore, some evidence suggests that the cerebral cortex may perform a general computation that can be generalized across modalities; thus, a generalized circuit that recapitulates this fundamental computation might serve as a useful replacement for multiple possible areas of cerebral cortex. It is possible that cortical prostheses that even partially restore cognitive function lost due to brain trauma or dementia could reduce the disabilities in patients. It would be beneficial if exogenously assembled elements could be made to function as cerebral cortex does, or if the remaining nondamaged portion of brain could respond to new inputs and perform useful functions that replace damaged portions. The ultimate goal of implantable neuronal networks will require insights from the developmental neurobiology of the cerebral cortex, as well as advances in a range of technologies necessary for creating brain networks, promoting neuronal connections, engineering stem cells to match host tissues, devising biodegradable materials as scaffolds for implantable networks, and delivering molecules to brain tissues.

Initial Challenges to Consider

• What kinds of disease conditions could be alleviated by a cerebral cortex prosthesis? Would different diseases require different approaches?

• How does the cerebral cortex function? What computation does it perform? Does the cerebral cortex perform a general computation or transformation of information that can be generalized across modalities, and can this be taken advantage of?

• What do you feel is the most promising general substrate for a cortical prosthetic?

    —tissue transplanted from analogous regions in the same or a different brain;

    — tissue grown externally and then implanted;

    —tissue already existing in the brain that could be coaxed to co-opt the function of interest; or

    —a nonbiological circuit substrate engineered to adopt the requisite function.

• Distinguish these potential avenues based on currently available technologies, cost of procedures, likelihood of success, and ethical considerations.

• A persistent problem with introducing new material into the brain is that the material is rejected by immune or neuroprotective responses. How might these responses be placated to facilitate the adoption of the new material by host brain?

• A further problem is that the substitute neural tissue may need to reasonably match the host tissue in order to function effectively. For example, the prosthesis may need to be primed to be responsive to specific activity levels, and its response properties and activity levels must in turn roughly correspond to those expected by their downstream projections. What functional properties are most critical for general functional integration, and how might these properties be imbued into the substitute neural tissue?

• Finally, the prosthetic must be structurally connected to and integrated with surrounding circuits. What treatments might facilitate this connectivity? Candidate treatments could operate on either the macroscopic level by promoting axonal outgrowth from one region to another, or on a more refined scale by fostering the development of individual local neuronal connections.

Initial References

Bradbury, E. J., and S. B. McMahon. 2006. Spinal cord repair strategies: Why do they work? Nature Reviews Neuroscience 7:644-653.

Gage, F. H. 2003. Brain, repair yourself. Scientific American 289:47-53.

George, P., A. Lyckman, D. LaVan, A. Hegde, Y. Liung, R. Avasare, C. Testa, P. Alexander, R. Langer, and M. Sur. 2005. Fabrication and biocompatibility of polypyrrole implants suitable for neural prostheses. Biomaterials 26:3511-3519.

Harel, N., and S. Strittmatter. 2006. Can regenerating axons recapitulate developmental guidance during recovery from spinal cord injury. Nature Reviews Neuroscience 7: 603-616.

Maher, M. P., J. Pine, J. Wright, and Y.-C. Tai. 1999. The neurochip: A new multielectrode device for stimulating and recording from cultured neurons. Journal of Neuroscience Methods 87:45-56.

Sur, M., and J. Rubenstein. 2005. Patterning and plasticity of the cerebral cortex. Science 310:805-810.

TASK GROUP SUMMARY

Summary written by:

Elizabeth ("Beth") Quill, Graduate Science Writing Student, Massachusetts Institute of Technology

Task group members:

• Dennis Barbour, Assistant Professor, Biomedical Engineering, Washington University in St. Louis

- Theodore Berger, David Packard Professor of Engineering; Director, Center for Neural Engineering, University of Southern California
- Kenneth C. Curley, Chief Scientist, U.S. Army Telemedicine and Advanced Technology Research Center
- James Fallon, Professor, Anatomy and Neurobiology, University of California, Irvine
- William Foster, Assistant Professor, Physics, The University of Houston
- William Heetderks, Director, Extramural Science Program, National Institute of Biomedical Imaging and Bioengineering, National Institutes of Health
- Pedro Irazoqui, Assistant Professor, Weldon School of Biomedical Engineering, Purdue University
- Kenneth Jaffe, Professor, Rehabilitation Medicine, Adjunct Professor, Pediatrics and Neurological Surgery, University of Washington School of Medicine; Editor in Chief, Archives of Physical Medicine and Rehabilitation
- David Mooney, Professor, Division of Engineering and Applied Sciences, Harvard University
- Isaac Mwase, Associate Professor of Philosophy and Bioethics, National Center for Bioethics, Tuskegee University
- Randolph Nudo, Director, Landon Center on Aging, and Professor, Molecular and Integrative Physiology, The University of Kansas Medical Center
- Cengiz Ozkan, Assistant Professor, Mechanical Engineering, University of California, Riverside
- Elizabeth ("Beth") Quill, Graduate Science Writing Student, Massachusetts Institute of Technology
- Molly Shoichet, Professor and Director, Undergraduate Collaborative Bioengineering, Canada Research Chair in Tissue Engineering, University of Toronto

Summary

Complicated problems often require new ways of thinking. And replacing cortical tissue, connecting it, and convincing it to work is about as complicated as they come. So, when neurosurgeons, neurobiologists, physicians, engineers, and a philosopher got together at the National Academies Keck *Futures Initiative* Conference in November, they began by brainstorming ways to think about the problem. "We all have different perspectives and will probably define the problem a bit differently," said Randolph Nudo, director of the Landon Center on Aging and professor of molecular and integrative physiology at the University of Kansas Medical Center. "I'd like to get a feeling for what people think our challenge is."

The Problem Defined

Ideas began to flow. Then came the questions. What types of tissue should be included? What kind brain damage should be considered? Who would the patients be? Should the solution be based on tissue growth or an implanted chip? Should growth or connectivity be the main concern? The conversation continued this way until David Mooney, professor in the Division of Engineering and Applied Sciences at Harvard University, suggested the group take a step back. "Right now we are talking about a number of things," he said. "The scope will fall from the definition of the problem."

Mooney's advice led the group to the drawing board, literally. James Fallon, professor of anatomy and neurobiology at the University of California, Irvine, grabbed a marker and began sketching arrows on the board in the front of the room to represent the feedback systems in the brain.

"Do we care about information that goes to the brain stem or spinal cord?" Fallon asked.

"Forget about it," replied Ted Berger, director of the Center for Neural Engineering at the University of Southern California.

"Do we need anything else?" Fallon asked.

"Just stop there; that is enough," Berger replied.

The diagram looked a little overwhelming but the exercise was instructive. And since Fallon accidentally used a Sharpie marker on the white board, the group could refer back to the diagram throughout the day. After a bit more discussion, a problem statement emerged. Such is the process of science.

Dennis Barbour, assistant professor of biomedical engineering at Washington University in St. Louis, wrote a possible statement on the board. "This is a problem statement," Barbour said. "Should this be our problem statement?" With a few word changes a specific but flexible definition of the problem took shape.

The group decided to focus on damage to the cerebral cortex, the outer surface of the brain responsible for reasoning, mood, and perception. Members also decided to limit the solution to severe and permanent damage. For this reason the solution would be most useful in situations where conventional treatment failed. A simple solution that could work for a number of types of damage would also be ideal. Fallon's arrows provided some first clues. And at the end of the first day the group had something to work with.

The Model

When the group reconvened, Barbour decided to take advantage of PowerPoint. Everyone could see the screen and he could easily pull up needed information. "This is a lot easier than messing around with the white board," Barbour said. Berger joked back, "Particularly because we can't erase it anymore." All kidding aside, the group had defined the problem, but what next? Pedro Irazoqui, assistant professor of biomedical engineering at Purdue University, said the next step was hiring graduate students. The group thought long and hard and decided that instead they needed to get back to work.

Vision could provide a good model to help solve the group's problem because damage to the visual cortex is localized and easy to test. In addition, the circuitry underlying the visual function in primates has been studied extensively, which could help successfully model some of this circuitry. The information passes for the most part in one direction. The group focused on central scotomas—blind spots sometimes caused by stroke. Berger had worked with a similar pathway in the hippocampus. "If you have to reproduce every connection in every single cell, you might as well go home," Berger said. "You have to approximate the problem with some smaller inputs and sample the outputs you simulate." He said the smallest details of what happens where are not necessarily important. Instead, the group needed to understand and re-create the signal. This, of course, would be no small task.

Berger encouraged the group to think of information traveling from point A to B to C. At each stage the information is processed in some way. If B is eliminated, researchers can measure the signals leaving A and entering C, and then they can develop a chip that replicates B's function. "It just does an input-output mapping," Berger said. "And if you don't like the model, you change what is inside there and you get a different one." By breaking the problem down into steps and by avoiding too many details, the group could move forward. Solutions began to emerge, a bit piecemeal, but by the final day they came together.

The Solutions

After agreeing that there was no perfect solution, the group decided to outline possible solutions. Bill Heetderks, director of the Extramural Science program at the National Institute of Biomedical Imaging and Bioengineering, supported this move. "It seems to me if you are buying stock where you don't know the result, you should diversify," he said. "The notion that we can put forth one solution is not realistic for what we know." Instead, the group began with two assumptions. All of the solutions involve artificial electronic circuits and all require cortical plasticity. The group stuck with the visual cortex as a model.

The first solution the group called the "electronic prosthesis." In this solution an artificial computational system on a microchip would replace the damaged tissue. Wires would connect the chip to inputs and outputs and the chip would serve the function of the damaged cortex. Electrodes would supply the signals. The second solution, called the "hybrid electronic neural prosthesis," would be similar except neurons instead of electrodes would interact with the chip.

But both these options present a number of challenges. "There is a significant problem with the interface," Nudo said. "We are talking about systems where we have cultured neurons growing on a substrate . . . but the neurons don't like the prosthetic environment." If a workable interface could be developed in the first case, the number and density of the electrodes would also need to be considered. And if the system worked, scientists would still need to model the inputs and outputs and have the computational power to make the process possible. In the case of the hybrid system, scientists would also have to learn to direct neuronal growth.

A third option would involve growing new cortical tissue and using the microchip to teach this tissue to serve the required function. The group called it a "de novo engineered neural circuitry prosthesis." And a fourth alternative would be to co-opt less important tissue in the brain and use a chip to train this region to serve the missing tissue's function. The third and fourth, called the "in situ cortical isograft prosthesis," would capitalize on circuitry that already exists. And both would mean the device could eventually be removed. "The brain could remodel over time," said William Foster, assistant professor of physics at the University of Houston.

But these solutions also present challenges. Both would still require a workable interface. And scientists would have to know how to train synaptic connections and train neurons to differentiate and to grow in the right places and in the right directions. Furthermore, in the case of the third solution, cortical tissue would have to be grown. Berger said this is a challenge, though material scientists are developing some scaffolding. "One of the problems is neurons can attach and grow nicely, but they grow in both directions," Berger said.

The Next Step

The group came to no consensus on the best first approach to test, and group members still had general concerns. Would unconsidered solutions be easier or safer? And is a general solution even possible? More research needed to be done in neurobiology, bio- and nanomaterials, tissue engineering, computer engineering, and computational physiological modeling to answer these questions. Still the group worked until the last minute, cross-examining their ideas and assumptions. "Is it OK to make bionic people?" asked Irazoqui. "What public policy changes would have to be made with cognitive enhancing abilities available?" continued Berger. After eight hours of discussion and a healthy amount of hand waving, the group had defined approaches and challenges associated with each.

In the United States 700,000 people have strokes each year and 1.7 million suffer from traumatic brain injury. A proportion of these lose important brain function, including function associated with sight, control of extremities, and language capacity. The group members certainly weren't ready to begin accepting volunteers for clinical trials, but they were able to integrate old ideas and develop new ones. And the product of their work proves that 15 interdisciplinary professionals committed to a problem can make progress.

Build a Smart Prosthesis That Will Grow with a Child (such as a Heart Valve or Cerebral Shunt, or a Self-Healing Prosthesis)

TASK GROUP DESCRIPTION

Pediatric Cardiac Valves

Background

The most common congenital valve problem in children is aortic stenosis (i.e., restricted aortic outflow). In the past, stenotic valves were commonly dilated with balloon catheters or surgically incised to increase the opening. Unfortunately, after balloon dilatation or surgery, valve integrity is compromised with significant leakage, which strains the left ventricle leading to dilation and dysfunction.

Replacement of an abnormal aortic valve in a small child is a unique challenge, particularly in sizing the new valve. There are no manufactured valves that perform well in very small children. The smallest successful artificial valve is roughly 17 millimeters in diameter, which infants with congenital aortic stenosis often cannot spatially accommodate. Enlargement of the aortic root can sometimes provide enough room to tolerate a 17 millimeter or 19 millimeter valve (using the Konno procedure) but not without consequence. Even with the Konno modification, implantation of a full adult-sized valve is impossible in very small children. Therefore, these pa-

15

tients will inevitably outgrow the implant and will require further surgery later in life.

In addition, mechanical valve substitutes also require lifelong protection against clotting with anticoagulant medications to prevent thrombus formation on the valve leaflets, which can cause strokes or lead to dysfunction of the valve. Implantations of animal tissue or xenograft valves avoid the need for anticoagulation but do not resolve this dilemma. Tissue valves are prone to premature calcification and degeneration in growing children. Even human homograft (cadaver) valves used in small infants tend to calcify before the patient reaches adulthood.

To overcome these significant problems with surgical treatment of congenital aortic valve disease, the Ross procedure was developed. In the Ross procedure the pulmonic valve is switched to the aortic position, where it continues to grow, and the pulmonic valve is replaced with a cadaveric homograft. This is the best long-term treatment for children with aortic valve and root abnormalities. The native tissue reconstruction provided by the Ross procedure also eliminates the burden and complications of anticoagulation. Moreover, the pulmonary autograft neither calcified nor degenerated over time in contradistinction to xenograft bioprosthesis.

A modified Ross autotransplant performed in concert with annular enlargement, the Konno-Ross, is performed by first harvesting additional muscle from the anterior right ventricular outflow tract as the autograft is procured. After removal of the diseased aortic valve, the aortic annulus is split open between the right and left coronary arteries. Then the pulmonic donor graft is sewn into this enlarged annulus, including the additional muscle skirt harvested with the autograft. The pulmonary homograft reconstruction of the right heart is purposely oversized to permit growth of the child and reduce the need for secondary operations. Although technically demanding, the use of the Ross operation in pediatric patients with aortic valve disease is clearly a major step forward in the surgical management of these patients.

Initial Challenges to Consider

•   Children who need a mitral valve replacement commonly receive a mechanical valve made of polymers or metals that are very durable. With a mechanical valve, anticoagulation is required chronically, and in a young child the valve would need replacement at least one time later in life as it becomes too small. Unlike the Ross procedure for the aortic valve, there are no similar procedures for the mitral valve.

• How can the atrial-ventricular valve be engineered to restore and maintain cardiac function? What will control the growth and development of the valve? Are there alternative ways in which the functional status of the valve can be monitored?

Vascular Grafts

Background

The replacement or repair of diseased vessels with natural synthetic vascular grafts has become a routine treatment for certain types of intravascular disease. In coronary bypass surgery the autologous saphenous vein remains the graft of choice for its nonthrombogenic flow surface, ability to be healed by the host, as well as its strength and elasticity. Development of a synthetic small diameter vascular graft has been largely unsuccessful. Moreover, for the pediatric population these grafts are fixed and do not conform to patient growth from childhood into adulthood. The unfortunate therapeutic strategy thus necessitates multiple surgeries.

Initial Challenges to Consider

Many laboratories are attempting to create an alternative to autologous veins for use in coronary artery bypass grafting and other shunt procedures. In general, researchers are either attempting to engineer nonthrombogenic synthetic materials for use as conduits or to tissue engineer living blood vessels from cells and scaffold.

One research tactic has been to create a three-dimensional construct from porous matrices (such as collagen, elastin, or polyglycolic acid), and seed them with cells. Some investigators re-create relevant biochemical and mechanical environments to allow endothelial smooth-muscle cells and fibroblasts to proliferate within an extracellular matrix under appropriate applied stresses. Another approach has been to create grafts from small intestine submucosa (SIS), which remodel into the tissue where they are implanted.

Can these or similar approaches be employed to create biologically compatible grafts that will not require lifelong anticoagulation and which will remodel to the demands of a growing patient? What approach would be best?

Initial References

Flanagan, T. C., and A. Pandit. 2003. Living artificial heart valve alternatives: A review. European Cells & Materials 6:28-45; discussion 45, Nov. 20.

Hoerstrup, S. P., A. Kadner, S. Melnitchouk, A. Trojan, E. Eid, J. Tracy, R. Sodian. J. F. Visjager, S. A. Kolb, J. Grunenfelder, G. Zund, and M. I. Turina. 2002. Tissue engineering of functional trileaflet heart valves from human marrow stromal cells. Circulation 106(12)(Suppl. 1):I143-I150.

Nemecek, S. 1995. Have a heart. Scientific American, June, p. 46.

Simon, P., M. T. Kasimir, G. Seebacher. G. Weigel, R. Ullrich, U. Salzer-Muhar, E. Rieder, and E. Wolner. 2003. Early failure of the tissue engineered porcine heart valve SYNERGRAFT in pediatric patients. European Journal of Cardio-Thoracic Surgery 23(6):1002-1006; discussion 1006, June.

Sutherland, F. W., and J. E. Mayer Jr. 2003. Ethical and regulatory issues concerning engineered tissues for congenital heart repair. Seminars in thoracic and cardiovascular surgery. Pediatric Cardiac Surgery Annual 6:152-163.

TASK GROUP SUMMARY

Summary written by:

Kate Fink, Graduate Student, Science Journalism, Boston University

Task group members:

- Donald Eigler, IBM Fellow, IBM Almaden Research Center
- Kate Fink, Graduate Student, Science Journalism, Boston University
- Steven Gard, Research Associate Professor, Physical Medicine and Rehabilitation, Northwestern University
- Jeremy L. Gilbert, Professor and Associate Dean for Research, Biomedical and Chemical Engineering, Syracuse University
- Irene W. Leigh, Ph.D., Professor, Department of Psychology, Gallaudet University
- Helen H. Lu, Assistant Professor, Biomedical Engineering, Columbia University
- Carlos Pena, Senior Science Policy Analyst, OC/OSHC, Food and Drug Administration, Health and Human Services
- Buddy Ratner, Director, University of Washington Engineered Biomaterials (UWEB); Professor, Bioengineering and Chemical Engineering, University of Washington

• Frances Richmond, Director, Regulatory Science Program, School of Pharmacy, University of Southern California
• Khaled Saleh, Associate Professor, Orthapedic Surgery; Division Head and Fellowship Director, Adult Reconstruction, University of Virginia

Summary

Human heart valves derived from the stem cells in a mother's amniotic fluid could be grown by scientists before a baby's birth, ready to repair heart defects when the child is born, reported scientists at November's American Heart Association meeting.[1]

A recent study in chickens revealed that vertebrates—including humans—may possess the genetic signals needed to regenerate limbs the way salamanders do. Researchers at the Salk Institute for Biological Studies stimulated the proper signals in a chick, inducing expression of the genes needed to grow back an amputated wing, according to an article published in *Genes and Development.*[2]

And *Outside Magazine* lists tissue engineering as number 70 on its December 2006 list of 100 of "the year's most important people, ideas, trends, and gear"—right between a Pro pogo stick and a scenic waterfall in Peru.[3]

The field is decidedly hot, but building a "smart" prosthetic that can grow with a child—the aim of this task group—represents a formidable challenge. Development of these prosthetics represents a field rich with potential, one that might take great advantage of the advances mentioned above. Yet, many gaps in our knowledge remain on the road to clinical use of such technology. The potential benefits make the trip worth traveling, however, and this task group concentrated on identifying the areas where we lack knowledge and how we might begin to bridge these gaps in understanding.

The additional issue of growth raises the degree of difficulty in creating prostheses for children, in addition to the scientific and technological challenges inherent in building any prosthesis—such as compatibility with the host, integration with host tissues, and control of the prosthesis. Growth, as the task group defined it, includes changes in size, performance of the prosthetic, rate of growth, and complexity—in terms of the child's changing cognitive, emotional and hormonal, behavioral, and biological state.

Charge to Task Group

The task of building a smart prosthesis to grow with a child encompasses a diverse array of scenarios—from heart valves to bones to blood vessels or bladders. Some examples of prostheses that grow with children already exist: An artificial femur can lengthen within a child's leg to keep pace with growth, expanding every one to two years via noninvasive stimulation controlled by a doctor.[4] Several children recently received laboratory-grown bladders built from their own cells.[5] Though, as these children grow no one can yet be certain how the bladders will grow and adjust within their changing bodies.

So many possibilities exist that the task group started to get a handle on the problem by categorizing examples of prosthetics that need to grow with children according to the degree of difficulty associated with developing them. The relatively easier end of the spectrum included bones and shunts to drain cerebrospinal fluid. Growing an entire limb or creating a device that requires an interface between brain and machine that must incorporate an element of cognitive development pose the most challenging problems. As the challenge increases, the group noted, so too does the need for interdisciplinary collaboration to address it. An orthopedic surgeon might develop an artificial bone that grows, but creating a prosthetic that interacts with a child's changing brain will require input from neurologists, neurosurgeons, engineers, materials scientists, and developmental psychologists. This stratification by difficulty of each task helped to identify the scope of challenges to address, and allowed the group to clearly see what thematic concerns spread across all of these specific cases.

Knowing what we don't know can be the key to heading in the right direction for the answer. The group focused much of its time on developing a taxonomy to use in thinking about how to develop a smart prosthetic to grow with a child.

Strategy

Making a prosthetic that can grow with a child requires many decisions. First, in the taxonomy developed by the task group a primary choice must be made between two general strategies: building the prosthetic using tissue engineering and regenerative medicine or using synthetic systems. Tissue engineering, such as that used to create the bladders already in use, might use a child's own cells to grow an organ outside of the body. A synthetic system could allow for preparation of a tissue—such as a heart valve—from artificial materials to be placed in the body during an emergency situation, when doctors and researchers do not have the time to grow one from a patient's own cells.

The next decision involves making control of the prosthetic active or passive. On the passive end of this continuum, the prosthetic would require no regulation by the child. The device's adaptation and growth with the child would be autoregulated. On the other end an active device would require a child to learn how to use it over time. A tertiary decision, control of the device, would require doctors and researchers to decide where the prosthetic's instructions came from. It might be controlled internally—carrying its roadmap for growth with it inside the body—perhaps in the timed release of certain growth factors. Or it might require a doctor to exert external control, such as radio frequency signals, to tell a prosthetic bone to lengthen a few centimeters every year or two, during a child's visit to the office.

Future Challenges

Researchers, doctors, and engineers must address several gaps in our knowledge to develop prosthetics that are smarter, more durable, and more accurate replications of natural tissues and organs. The task group identified several areas, including longevity, growth boundaries, and exploiting developmental biology, that present challenges unique to prosthetics intended for growing children.

The longevity of prosthetics in children must exceed that of any available to date. Adult patients receiving hip replacements today often outlive these artificial joints. A child's prosthetic must survive nearly a lifetime—70, 80, or over 90 years.

The growth boundaries on a child's prosthetic warrant thoughtful consideration: It must grow to the correct size while maintaining function and keeping pace with the child's growth but must also cease growth and segue into a "dynamic endstate"—a state, perhaps no longer physically growing but continuing to respond, adapt, and communicate with the body around it.

The ability of a prosthetic to work with a child's own developing brain or limbs might offer a meaningful advantage. Though creating a prosthetic for a child presents unique challenges, it also provides the opportunity to capitalize on the unique complement of growth factors and plasticity within a child's cells and tissues. But prosthetics can take advantage of this natural milieu only if the most advantageous window of time is precisely identified.

Bioethical, economic, and regulatory concerns also represent overarching issues that will infuse the decisions made in the course of developing these prosthetics for children.

Task Group Recommendations

Considering these gaps in current knowledge and the highly interdisciplinary nature of the work required to develop smart prosthetics to grow with a child, this task group recommended a future workshop with three general goals: building an initial plan for the immediate next steps required for research to move forward; establishing a calendar of attainable goals— which prosthetics for children are likely to be achievable within five years, ten years; and building of interdisciplinary teams amongst those at the fore-front—those in fields such as prosthetic research, developmental biology, tissue engineering, electrical engineering, surgery, and clinical medicine. The workshop, suggested this task group, might be most productive if organized into working groups based on specific prosthetic projects, such as heart valves, bladders, or legs.

One member of the group, Jeremy Gilbert of the Biomedical and Chemical Engineering Department at Syracuse University, said, "Clearly nature has worked out these mechanisms in exquisite detail." Now it's our turn to figure them out.

Notes

1. Scientific Sessions Daily News. 2006. Stem cell research takes promising new directions. 2006. American Heart Association, Nov. 15. Online at http://www.sessionsdailynews.com/wednesday.html#story4, accessed 1/3/2007. Wall Street Journal. 2006. Scientists grow heart valves employing amniotic stem cells. Nov. 16, p. D4.

2. Kawakami, Y., C. R. Esteban, M. Raya et al. 2006. Wnt/β-catenin signaling regulates vertebrate limb regeneration. Genes & Development 20:3232-3237.

3. Outside Magazine. 2006. The O List Outside One Hundred. Dec., p. 112-138.

4. Memorial Sloan-Kettering. n.d. Expandable prosthesis. Online at http://www.mskcc.org/mskcc/html/11953.cfm, accessed 1/3/07.

5. Atala, A., S. B. Bauer, S. Soker, J. J. Yoo, and A. B. Retik. 2006. Tissue engineered autologous bladders for patients needing cystoplasty. The Lancet 367(9518): 1241-1246.

Develop a Smart Prosthetic That Can Learn Better and/or Faster

TASK GROUP DESCRIPTION

Background

Even though prosthetics have come a long way since they have emerged, functional limitations and challenges of directly and reliably controlling them still makes artificial prostheses less than optimal for the satisfactory performance of everyday tasks of amputees. The challenges are mainly due to the range of motions required for satisfactory performance, which calls for a highly complex prosthetic mechanism to impart movements and a complex control interface to communicate with the prosthetic device.

Research performed over the past decade has led to the refinement of prosthetic materials. Materials that are capable of withstanding the physical and mechanical demands of the prostheses to a great extent are now available. Also, recent advances in bioengineering are greatly helping to develop robotic systems that could mechanically mimic many of the functions of the extremities.

However, to efficiently use a functional prosthetic much more control over prostheses is needed. Even though myoelectric prostheses have better control over body-powered prostheses, these devices involve a steep learning curve for the patients to gain conscious control over the weak electric signals. The finest approach to achieve full control of the prosthetic by the patient is by turning the thought process in the brain into actual physical movements of the prostheses using direct neural interfaces.

Initial Challenges to Consider

Several challenges remain unresolved to develop a practical interactive hybrid brain machine interface (HBMI) to control a prosthetic in real time.

• To control prostheses using HBMI real-time sampling and processing of large-scale brain activity is needed. This calls for the development of novel methods for measuring large-scale brain activity, learning how to sample and decode motor signals and how to feed them into prostheses to mimic the required movement, new techniques for microstimulating neuronal tissue, developments in microchip design, nano- and microfabrication techniques, and further developments in robotics.

• Lack of sensory feedback is another key limitation that seriously hinders the ability of the prosthesis to respond to external environment. The sensory feedback is highly essential to establish a closed control loop between brain and artificial prostheses and is also a great tool to help the patient to learn how to use HBMI's. However, this needs understanding of where and how to stimulate the sensory nervous system to reproduce the signals that an organ sends to sensory cortex.

• Materials integration is also needed. Interface implants need to be designed that can integrate with host tissue to obviate the need for frequent replacement.

Initial References

Abbot, A. 2006. Neuroprosthetics: In search of the sixth sense. Nature 442:125-127.
Biddiss, E., and T. Chau. 2006. Electroactive polymeric sensors in hand prostheses: Bending response of an ionic polymer metal composite. Medical Engineering & Physics 28: 568-578.
Chapin, J. K., and K. A. Moxon, eds. 2000. *Neural Prostheses for Restoration of Sensory and Motor Function*. Boca Raton: CRC.
Nicolelis, M. A. L. 2001. Actions from thoughts. Nature 409:403-407.

TASK GROUP SUMMARY

Summary written by:

Wendi Zongker, Graduate Student, Grady College of Journalism and Mass Communication Department, The University of Georgia

Task group members:

- James Abbas, Co-Director, Center for Adaptive Neural Systems, The Biodesign Institute
- Farid Amirouche, CEO and President, Ortho Sensing Technologies
- Bradford Bennett, Assistant Professor of Research, Orthopaedic Surgery; and Research Director, Motion Analysis and Motor Performance Laboratory, University of Virginia
- Nancy Byl, Professor and Chair, Physical Therapy and Rehabilitation Science Department, University of California, San Francisco
- Jose Luis Contreras-Vidal, Associate Professor of Kinesiology, Bioengineering and Neuroscience Program, University of Maryland
- Michael Dorman, Professor, Speech and Hearing Science, Arizona State University
- Gary K. Fedder, Howard M. Wilkoff Professor of Electrical and Computer Engineering and Robotics; Director, Institute for Complex Engineered Systems, Carnegie Mellon University
- Brent Gillespie, Assistant Professor, Mechanical Engineering, University of Michigan
- Anne Heberger, Research Associate, National Academies Keck *Futures Initiative*
- Hod Lipson, Assistant Professor, Mechanical and Aerospace Engineering, Cornell University
- Yoky Matsuoka, Associate Professor, Computer Science and Engineering, University of Washington
- Michael Merzenich, Francis Sooy Professor of Otolaryngology, Keck Center for Integrative Neurosciences, University of California, San Francisco, School of Medicine
- Santa Ono, Vice Provost and Deputy Provost, Emory University
- Kevin Otto, Assistant Professor, Weldon School of Biomedical Engineering and Biological Sciences, Purdue University

- Blake Wilson, Senior Fellow, RTI International
- Wendi Zongker, Graduate Student, Grady College of Journalism and Mass Communication Department, The University of Georgia

Summary

Doctors, scientists, researchers, engineers, CEOs, and even a provost traveled from all over the United States to put their different disciplines aside and work together for a common cause. These men and women traveled to the National Academies Keck *Futures Initiative* Conference held November 8-11, 2006, in Irvine, California, to discuss the future of prosthetics research. Attendees were divided into 11 groups, each with a different task to tackle and only three days and eight hours in which to accomplish that objective. Task group 3 was faced with the challenge of developing a "smart" prosthetic that can learn better and or faster.

What Is Learning?

It depends on what you mean by "learn."

That's what members of this task group identified as the starting point for three days of discussion about developing a smart prosthetic that can learn better and or faster. After a lengthy discussion, members of our group settled on one definition with two components. The first definition postulates that a device has a built-in predictive model that generates output depending on what information is fed into it. This is possible due to a feedback loop, which allows the model to act differently depending on what its previous actions have accomplished. The second definition defines learning as the act of organizing, or reorganizing, neural circuits so one can successfully interpret information and/or external signals and respond appropriately.

What Are the Challenges of This Task?

After much discussion about the purpose of a smarter prosthetic device, and about what it should and should not be designed to do, our group listed challenges that must be conquered to make it learn faster and better. These include developing a device that can remember what it's done and analyze how well its actions worked, which implies having recording capacity. The patient's brain is an integral part of the feedback loop that will help the device learn, and much less is known about this than about high-tech materials and robotics for prosthetic devices.

How Can We Promote Learning?

As the first day of discussion drew to a close, our group was focused on this question: What strategies best promote learning in both the patient and the prosthetic device? Participants agreed that motivation, repetition, progression, surprise, feedback, reward, and attention all promote learning, and they resolved to figure out which of these can be automated to maximize learning by client and machine.

Day 2

On the second day of the conference, our group had only two densely packed hours to solidify our definition of learning, consider how brain and machine should share the learning, begin considering what different customers will require of their prosthetic device, and decide what will be required to accomplish our assigned task.

After much discussion, the group agreed that learning is the method of reorganizing human neural circuits in the prosthetic device to interpret signals and generate cognitive/motor outputs. As circuits are reorganized, internal predictive models are adjusted and the planning and control of actions change. This happens on both the human and machine sides of the transaction, and the two collaborate and interact as they gain experience. The learning is ongoing and can result in bad learning or learning the wrong things.

The discussion quickly turned to the wisdom of trying to develop the smartest possible prosthetic that would shoulder most of the responsibility for translating thought into action. Some participants thought it would be ideal to have a device that became increasingly competent with experience and over time permitted the brain to become relatively "dumb." Others argued that it would be better to have the prosthetic back off over time, letting the human brain eventually do almost everything. If we can determine a way to connect the prosthetic to the human brain with enough connections, the prosthetic can become like a real limb—or dumb. This preferred option is unlikely to occur in the initial design, therefore, rather than beginning with a dumb prosthetic, smarts will need to be built into the device to interpret the limited transfer of information between the prosthetic and the human brain. Abbas summed it up by stating that "we want a prosthetic that is smart enough to do some of the job but not smart enough to do everything."

The discussions between developing a dumb prosthetic and a smart prosthetic included an idea among members of the group to develop a device that begins with reduced degrees of freedom, enabling simple operation by the user. Over time and with learning, complexity of the device will increase by releasing, or increasing, the degrees of freedom of operation as the user learns to use the prosthetic. This method of operation parallels how a human initially learns to use a motor task. A baby learning to walk looks stiff and unsure, as there are reduced degrees of freedom. As the baby grows and learns the skill of walking involves more degrees of freedom and therefore looks more fluid and smooth.

The group discussed various tasks that the prosthetic device should be able to do, which led them to consider how customer requirements will vary. The prosthetic will only be as good as its capacity to satisfy individual users, they decided, and one person might want to play basketball while another would be more than satisfied to simply walk again.

Day 3

On day three the group defined learning issues for the client, the prosthetic device, and the training program, which includes hardware and software.

For the client, learning issues include training strategies with neurophysiologic foundations, providing sensory stimuli, and monitoring the learning progress. Learning issues of the prosthetic device include machine learning, sensors, and interface. The learning issues of the training program consist of progressive challenges and performance metrics.

In the wake of traumatic injury or illness that make a prosthetic limb necessary, patients mainly want to overcome pain and disability and regain some measure of independence and mobility. They expect to get better, but adapting to a prosthetic device is a lengthy and difficult process. To succeed, group members agreed that patients need to be motivated and need to be rewarded for progress. The learning will be biochemical and genetic and will involve active exploration and repetition in the form of progressive challenges. For learning to occur in the client there must be a realistic delineation of expectations and the client must also be able to adhere to a training regimen. Exploiting brain plasticity and richness of the interface between human nervous system and machine are also key issues to explore when dealing with learning occurring in the client.

Knowledge and/or technology gaps exist in regard to learning occurring with the client. These gaps include the know-how to transmit information to and from the brain, specifics regarding sensory and motor representations used in the brain, mechanisms of plasticity, and how to maximally exploit the plasticity.

The key features of the newly developed smart prosthesis should include the basic functions of safety, consistency in performance, reliability of use, and independence of use. The device should also have a bidirectional information flow between the user, or the human brain, and the prosthesis. There must also be an ability to provide rich sensory information, such as force, posture, velocity, temperature, vibration, time, and direction, and the device should also integrate the sensory information with motor outputs. The device must be dynamically adaptive to the client and incorporate contextual information flow and should employ multiple motor outputs to enable a rich repertoire of tasks. This involves gradually enabling the degrees of freedom, as discussed earlier, and the complexity, as well as enabling posture balance, stability, and movement. A vital element of the device is a high-fidelity interface that can imply dumb prosthesis when operating with an enabled brain. The device will incorporate the ability of "amazondotcomification," or the capability to learn what the user wants and/or needs. High bandwidth and versatility is another key feature. Finally, this device must be able to anticipate and inhibit decrements in the interface, for example, scar formation.

The group identified knowledge and/or technology gaps that inhibit the development of these key features in the prosthetic device. For instance, there is a need for biomorphic sensor/actuators to ensure compatibility with neural representations. Also, to create this device we must know how to maintain and improve performance based on interface. The group decided that task groups 4 and 6 would address this need for further research (see the *Brain Interfacing with Materials* and *Structural Tissue Interfaces* sections for more information on these groups). Research is necessary to find out how to detect and communicate user intent and motor commands and to establish machine learning techniques that are appropriate for real time adaptation. Our group also decided that there is a need for research on redundancy of learning and how to exploit it for versatility and efficiency.

The training programs employed must be fun, exciting, engaging, and easy to use to help promote learning by the user. They should have a design that is based on principles of cognitive neuroscience. Repetition is needed while also incorporating progressive challenges. Also at issue is the quality of information involved with these training programs and the immediate feedback in regard to reward and errors. These programs must be task specific and client specific and include the ability to be modified by the trainer. The method of training should also include practice spaced over time and should be available and accessible to the client.

Knowledge and/or technology gaps in creating the ideal training program include the current inability to identify intermediate performance and neurophysiological milestones. There is also no way to determine the individuality of minimal detectable differences or the know-how to customize the prosthetic device for a specific user group that may have certain needs based on age, gender, or culture.

After laying out key features and issues and determining the necessary knowledge and existing technology gaps to make these ideas a reality, our group moved on to prioritize the research needs and lay out a research agenda for the future. These research priorities were divided into the client, prosthetic device, and training program groups.

Research is necessary to determine how the brain learns to handle rich sensory inputs as well as how the brain translates user intent to motor action for increasingly sophisticated function. To develop this prosthetic device, research must be completed to determine a way to access user intent and then utilize that access effectively. The idea of machine learning in a co-adaptive setting must also be explored. In regard to the training programs, research should and must be conducted to learn how to maximize progressive learning.

Brain Interfacing with Materials: Recording and Stimulation Electrodes

TASK GROUP DESCRIPTION

Background

A new view in systems neuroscience is that variability of spikes is centrally coordinated and that this brain-generated ensemble pattern in cortical structures is itself a potential source of cognition. Large-scale recordings from neuronal ensembles are needed for testing this theoretical framework. Most thought-controlled brain-machine interface (BMI) devices are also based on such invasive techniques. Ideally, feedback signals from BMI devices should also be utilized to directly alter firing patterns of central neurons.

Action potentials produce large transmembrane potentials in the vicinity of their somata that can be measured by placing a conductor in close proximity to a neuron. A cylinder with a radius 150 μm contains up to 1000 neurons in the cortex. The use of two or more recording sites allows for the triangulation of the position of the neurons because the amplitude of the recorded spike is a function of the distance between the neuron and the electrode.

Initial Challenges to Consider

Currently, there is a large gap between the number of routinely recorded and theoretically recordable neurons. An ideal electrode has a very small volume, so that tissue injury is minimized, and has a large number of recording sites for monitoring many neurons simultaneously. Micro-electro-mechanical system based devices can reduce the technical limitations inherent in wire electrodes, because with the same amount of tissue displacement the number of monitoring sites can be substantially increased. Furthermore, multiple sites can be arranged over a longer distance, thus allowing for the simultaneous recording of neuronal activity in the various cortical layers.

Progress in large-scale recording of neuronal activity depends on the development of three critical components:

1. Neuron-electrode interface for long-term recording and stimulation;
2. Spike sorting/identification of parallel spike trains; and
3. Extraction of the "neuronal code."

In addition to increasing the numbers of recording sites, on-chip amplification, filtering, and time-division multiplexing will dramatically decrease the number of wires between the brain and electronic equipment by directly feeding the multiplexed digital signal into a computer processor. Programmed microstimulation through the recording sites and potentially real-time signal processing will not only facilitate basic research but is also a prerequisite for efficient, fully implantable neural prosthetic devices.

Initial References

Buzsaki, G. 2004. Large-scale recording of neuronal ensembles. Nature Neuroscience 7(5):446-451.

Donoghue, J. P. 2002. Connecting cortex to machines: Recent advances in brain interfaces. Nature Neuroscience 5(Suppl.):1085-1088.

Harris, K. D., J. Csicsvari, H. Hirase, G. Dragoi, and G. Buzsaki. 2003. Organization of cell assemblies in the hippocampus. Nature 424 :552-556.

Henze, D. A., Z. Borhegyi, J. Csicsvari, A. Mamiya, K. D. Harris, and G. Buzsaki. 2000. Intracellular features predicted by extracellular recordings in the hippocampus in vivo. Journal of Neurophysiology 84: 390-400.

McNaughton, B. L., J. O'Keefe, and C. A. Barnes. 1983. The stereotrode: A new technique for simultaneous isolation of several single units in the central nervous system from multiple unit records. Journal of Neuroscience Methods 8:391-397.

Olsson, R. H. III, D. L. Buhl, M. N. Gulari, G. Buzsaki, and K. D. Wise. 2003. A silicon microelectrode array for simultaneous recording and stimulation in the hippocampus of free moving rats and mice. IEEE Engineering in Medicine and Biology 22:1968-1671.

Wise, K. D., and K. Najafi. 1991. Microfabrication techniques for integrated sensors and microsystems. Science 254:1335-1342.

TASK GROUP SUMMARY—GROUP 1

(Due to the popularity of this topic, two groups explored this topic. Please be sure to review the second write-up, which immediately follows this one.)

Summary written by:

Megan Chao, Graduate Student in Broadcast Journalism, Annenberg School for Communication, University of Southern California

Task group members:

- Ravi Bellamkonda, Professor, Biomedical Engineering, Georgia Institute of Technology
- Megan Chao, Graduate Student in Broadcast Journalism, Annenberg School for Communication, University of Southern California
- Elias Greenbaum, Corporate Fellow, Chemical Sciences Division, Oak Ridge National Laboratory
- William Hammack, Professor, Chemical and Biomolecular Engineering, University of Illinois at Urbana-Champaign
- Kendall Lee, Assistant Professor of Neurosurgery, Physiology, and Biomedical Engineering, Neurosurgery Department, Mayo Clinic, Rochester
- Pedram Mohseni, Assistant Professor, Electrical Engineering and Computer Science, Case Western Reserve University
- Vivian Mushahwar, Assistant Professor and AHFMR Scholar, Biomedical Engineering and Center for Neuroscience, University of Alberta
- Richard Normann, Professor, Bioengineering Department, University of Utah
- Matthew O'Donnell, Dean, College of Engineering, University of Washington
- Joseph Pancrazio, Program Director, Repair and Plasticity Cluster Department, Division of Extramural Research, National Institute of Neurological Disorders and Stroke, National Institutes of Health

• Aristides Requicha, Gordon Marshall Chair in Engineering, Computer Science Department, University of Southern California
• Heinz Wässle, Professor, Doctor, Max-Planck-Institut

Summary

The use of penetrating electrode arrays provides unprecedented access to individual or small groups of neurons in forming a basic foundation for neuroprosthetic applications. In his introduction, group leader Ravi Bellamkonda addressed the importance of prosthetics and the use of electrode arrays at the interface between the brain and external electronics. Essentially, the promise of neuroprosthetics is the improvement of quality of life in persons with sensory or motor deficits caused by disease or injury to the nervous system.

Applications utilized by electrode arrays include, but are not limited to, recording signals from neurons and stimulation of neuronal activity. An invasive electrode array provides the interface between the brain and the prosthetic, and successful implantation and integration may result in full restoration of neurological function. An example of cochlear implants was provided, which currently employ an electrode array to transmit impulses from a stimulator to various regions of the auditory nerve. Also, individuals who experience profound levels of blindness may be able to restore some functional vision by way of a cortical-based visual neuroprosthesis, a research interest of group member Richard Normann.

Recordings can sometimes be made over significant periods of time, but in many instances the quality of those recordings deteriorates over a six-month time frame. Working group members identified the following as a major challenge for brain interfacing with materials: creation of penetrating electrode arrays that can reliably record or stimulate neuronal activity for longer than one year without jeopardizing the biocompatibility of the implant.

Mechanisms of Electrode Failure

Understanding the importance of electrode arrays in neuroprosthetic applications first requires recognition of the mechanisms of electrode failure. Group members agreed that failure is not limited to the physical construction of the electrode itself, but may also be the result of other factors, such as implantation, scarring, or micromotion.

The implantation of an electrode array runs the risk of cell and/or tissue damage, either vascular or neuronal. Group member Kendall Lee discussed deep brain stimulation for Parkinson's disease, as an example. There is a 2 percent to 3 percent chance of brain hemorrhage in the implantation process, as it involves advancing the electrode through the brain to the target site where nerve signals generate tremors or other symptoms associated with the disease. Although considered safe and effective, he said that improvements in targeting may further lower the risk.

The formation of scar tissue around an electrode array unquestionably contributes to the failure of the electrode in its ability to accurately collect and transmit neuronal signals. Scarring is a result of the body's natural wound repair process, occurring as a result of implantation, and the physiology of scar tissue may make for diminished electrode functionality. Identifying whether a correlation exists between scarring and failure, and whether a scar is electrically insulating may bridge a gap in understanding electrode failure. Micromotion, or the movement of the electrode away from its targeted active site, may be a contributing factor to scarring as well.

With respect to physical properties of electrode arrays, materials may induce biofouling of electrical contacts between the electrode array and the neuron with which it is interacting, meaning that a contamination linked to protein deposition from brain interstitial tissue or even microbial activity may occur. A high-charge injection may also cause the device to fail.

Parameters

In the construction of short- and long-term solutions to the aforementioned predicaments, group members established engineering and process parameters, as they were necessary in defining the capabilities and limitations of a system. The materials used to construct the electrode arrays may potentially be influenced by the electrode geometry, the ratio of stress it can withstand within the targeted tissue, or tools used for implantation.

What Constitutes "Smartness"?

Before addressing short- and long-term solutions to the task at hand, group members paused to define what exactly a smart prosthetic would be. In order for a material interface to the brain to be considered smart, it would need to be adaptive and sensitive to its dynamic environment. It may include properties of self-healing and/or self-repair, and have feedback or feed-forward controls. Suggestions from group members included designing an electrode to move autonomously or to be able to dynamically sense the local environment and release drugs to mitigate damage.

The group recognized the cost associated with smartness: Smartness requires complexity, and the potential cost of making the device too smart would be an increased chance of failure. Until there is a clear understanding of the mechanism of neurite extension and growth, in conjunction with knowledge of neuron function, a smart neuroprosthetic will remain a concept of the future.

Potential Short-Term Approaches

Group members decided on the second day of collaboration that a working timeline over 10 years would be considered in identifying a potential solution short-term. A short-term approach would be able to utilize present knowledge and/or present research data in the construction of new and improved neuroprosthetic systems.

An active exploration of scarring and its contribution to electrode failure, either by immunohistological techniques, state-of-the-art in vivo molecular imaging, or impedance spectroscopy, would provide a more detailed understanding of the mechanisms with which they fail. The group also identified the need for quantitative assessment of micromotion and a correlation with neural recording stability.

The group members speculated on potential solutions to fixing mechanisms of electrode failure. These included the development of electrodes with smaller cross-sectional areas, like implantable quantum dots with nanowire connections. There was also recognition that there may be considerable benefits in usage of other materials beyond silicon and microwires. Advances in biomaterial research could result in electrode materials that match the compliance of brain tissue.

The smaller size of the electrode inherently reduces implantation risks, but achieving electrical interfaces become an issue. Group member Pedram Mohseni suggested wireless interfacing, as the technology is highly prevalent in today's society. The development of a wireless communication system to power the electrode, as well as allowing it to receive and transmit signals, would naturally be the next step. Also, proper packaging of the electrode for implantation, perhaps by hermetic sealing, is vital to the success of the implanted electrode array.

Potential Long-Term Approaches

The group maintained a "blue sky" mentality as they considered long-term solutions. Identifying whether or not fundamental differences existed between tissue responses to recording and stimulating electrodes posed the challenge of whether there needed to be completely different strategies for designing electrodes or electrode arrays for recording and stimulation.

While there was a consensus in the necessity to make smaller high-density electrodes, group members decided it was just as important to consider biology in the actual architecture and design. This means utilizing present working knowledge of specific system functions and physiologies in the creation, which may become known as application-specific electrode arrays.

As far as implantation is concerned, it may be feasible to consider the development of methods to make tissues surrounding the implant site more permissive to the implant. Also, using nanomaterials in the construction of the electrode may significantly reduce resistance and enhance the biocompatibility of electrode surfaces.

Once the electrode is implanted, a source of power is necessary for function, and then a network can be built throughout the body to power electrodes and interact with arrays.

The group also considered the option of developing an alternative, nonelectrical means of interfacing with the peripheral or central nervous systems. Harnessing light or using molecular photovoltaic structures may provide other avenues for stimulation, while neurotransmitters as well as field potentials may be an alternative for sensing.

What All of This Means for Smart Prosthetics

The short- and long-term possibilities for the advancement of neuroprosthetics ultimately bring into context where the future of smart prosthetics may be. Continuing from the earlier discussion about what constitutes "smart," group members brainstormed examples of smart interfaces including encapsulating materials that react to emerging scar formation, the autopositioning of individual electrodes for optimizing signal acquisition, and microfluidics for injecting materials to make the tissue more permissive.

Interdisciplinary research in smart prosthetics will essentially evolve better devices and systems for improvement in the quality of life. As an example, utilizing biology to interact with biology to create the bio-based/ hybrid interface may be the smart prosthetic of tomorrow. Instead of having solid electrode arrays as we do now, it may be possible to create self-inserting bioelectrodes that grow into the tissue with minimal issues in biocompatibility. For instance, this may be done by sowing a feeder layer of genetically modified neurons onto the surface of the cortex, from which dendrites and axons grow into brain tissue. Synaptic connections are made and can thus "tap" brain signals. Electrical activity within this feeder layer could then be recorded. It may also be possible to create optically based interfaces by utilizing the work of group member Elias Greenbaum, who works in extracting Photosystem I of green plants and inserting them into excitable cells. He said that Photosystem I is a robust system and works quickly by capturing photon energy to do reduction-oxidation reactions.

As with all biological, chemical and engineering processes, it comes down to feasibility and practicality of the proposed solutions. How would neurite in-growth and targeting be controlled? How would reliable and functional synapses be formed and how would we promote that action? How would access be provided for the tissue-engineered interface? Would they be electrical or optical? And could the concept of creating the functional smart prosthetic lie in biomimetic interfacing? With all of these questions in mind and after almost eight hours of collaboration, group members were excited to be on the brink of developing the next successful smart prosthetic.

TASK GROUP SUMMARY—GROUP 2

(Due to the popularity of this topic, two groups explored this topic. Please be sure to review the first write-up, which immediately precedes this one.)

Summary written by:

Edyta Zielinska, Graduate Science Writing Student, New York University

Task group members:

• Orlando Auciello, Materials Science Department, Argonne National Laboratory

• Scott Beardsley, Assistant Professor, Biomedical Engineering Department, Marquette University
• Chet de Groat, Professor of Pharmacology, University of Pittsburgh
• Aparna Gupta, Assistant Professor, Decision Sciences and Engineering Systems, Rensselaer Polytechnic Institute
• Gareth Hughes, Senior Engineer Biomedical, Zyvex Corporation
• Themis Kyriakides, Assistant Professor, Biomedical Engineering and Pathology, Yale University
• David Martin, Professor, Materials Science and Engineering Department, The University of Michigan
• Karen Moxon, Associate Professor, School of Biomedical Engineering, Drexel University
• Alan Porter, NAKFI Evaluation Coordinating Consultant, and Technology Policy and Assessment Center Department, Georgia Tech
• Gerwin Schalk, Research Scientist IV, Brain-Computer Interface R&D Program, Wadsworth Center, New York State Department of Health
• Elmar T. Schmeisser, Neurophysiology & Cognitive Neurosciences, U.S. Army Research Office
• Bruce C. Wheeler, Professor and Interim Head, Bioengineering Department, University of Illinois
• Edyta Zielinska, Graduate Science Writing Student, New York University

Summary

Using technology to restore lost functions of hearing, vision, movement, scientists are working to make reality out of what was once considered within the realm of miracles.

One of the first success stories in this field of bionics, or neural prosthetics, is the cochlear implant. For those with severe hearing impairment it brings the ability to hear sound again. The technology is based on the simple idea that by stimulating the auditory nerve with electrical signals from a microphone, a person can understand those signals and hear again. Thousands of people around the world have been surgically implanted with this technology and are capable of hearing again, proof of the remarkable concept that electronics can communicate directly with human nerves. Now researchers are attempting to move from the auditory system to more complex systems, such as vision, and thereby developing new technology that could restore a greater variety of abilities.

The scientists in this arena generally don't talk about the miraculous nature of their research. Rather, they discuss the very concrete problems of actually making the devices work. One question at the very center of this endeavor is what happens when hard and rigid devices physically touch the soft, ever changing and adapting human tissue. How can the device be affected, and how does the tissue react? Despite much research, there is still much debate surrounding these questions, especially when the tissue in question is brain tissue.

A diverse group of 12 researchers, engineers, and funders convened as part of the Fourth Annual National Academies Keck *Futures Initiative* in Irvine, California, to discuss this problem, central to the future of many critical technologies. The group was charged with discussing how the brain interacts with materials. It soon became clear that the central and unavoidable first problem was why electrodes implanted in the brain often stop performing their function after a period of time.

Solving this problem of limited robustness of the interface between electronics and the nervous system could greatly advance the science of bionics. Finding ways to make the electrode work longer in the brain would help advance technologies like the retinal implant (bionic vision) and cochlear implant (already available bionic hearing). Longer lasting brain electrodes could also improve the electrical brain stimulation systems, like those used to relieve the tremors of Parkinson's disease, as well as electrodes that pick up the brain's signals and help paralyzed patients control electronic devices just by thinking.

Researchers working on brain implantation in animals have been frustrated by the problem of why electrodes don't work consistently for sustained periods of time. Researchers have observed that over time, some implanted electrodes stop receiving signals from the surrounding neurons. "The problem is that we don't know why it doesn't work," said Karen Moxon, associate professor of biomedical engineering at Drexel University. However, she and others doubted that it was a failure of the electrode itself. Her laboratory had taken an electrode that failed in one animal, cleaned it, and implanted it again in a new animal. "The electrode would work fine," she said.

If the electrode isn't broken and the brain isn't broken that leaves the area of space where the two touch. The problem appears to hinge exactly on "the mysterious 100 μm of space" surrounding the electrode, as Bruce Wheeler, professor and interim head of the bioengineering department at the University of Illinois, put it. The group floated a number of ideas of what might be happening in that area. David Martin, professor at the materials science and engineering department of the University of Michigan provided several images of his work that showed the area around the electrode in an experimental animal stained for neurons and for cells that typically respond to injury to the brain (e.g., astrocytes and microglia). In one image the neurons cleared away from the area surrounding the electrode, and in another image, astrocytes crowded in close. While it was unclear whether the scarring caused by the brain's reaction caused the failure, there was agreement that this space between the neurons and the electrode would somehow need to be bridged.

Another issue was what Martin called, "the fork in the Jell-O problem." The microscopic wiggling of a hard metallic device against the mushy brain tissue could either change the position of the electrode, or cause continual inflammation in the area.

Soon the real brainstorming of this lively group began. The "what about a thing that does this" and "what if we do that" ideas started flying across the room. Every new suggestion was returned with another even more fantastic sounding solution: "What if we coated the electrode with chemicals that would suppress the inflammation that might be causing the inflammation and scarring?" "What if we made an electrode that would deliver those chemicals to the area as they were needed?" "You can't deliver a drug forever, plus there's the question of toxicity." "What if we could make electrodes grow wires deeper into the brain, past the area of interface?"

But even as the ideas got more creative, it was clear that these scientists weren't simply daydreaming, but that these were actual technologies and techniques that were currently in development in their labs. Some of them already exist, while others were on their way to being created.

What if we could make an electrode that had the ability to scrape away the scars as they formed: "an in situ cleaning tool," said Gareth Hughes, senior biomedical engineer at Zyvex Corporation. To this seemingly wild suggestion Themis Kyriakides, assistant professor of biomedical engineering and pathology at Yale University, replied with a straight face, "We're working on it."

To address the problem of the neurons that were retreating away from the electrode, two approaches were suggested. There was the "Hansel and Gretel approach," as Martin put it, which was to attract the neurons to the electrodes by candy coating them with chemicals that neurons could not resist drawing toward. The other method was to bring the technology out to the neurons themselves. Tiny nanowires were sent out from the electrode, past the problematic 100 μm, to make connections with neurons that could still provide a signal.

An alternative version of the nanowire approach was proposed by Chet de Groat, professor of pharmacology at the University of Pittsburgh. Perhaps the surface of the electrode could be engineered in such a way to improve the electrical and mechanical interactions with the tissue, either by using stem cells or genetically engineered cells. "We could make these cells sniffers," said de Groat, using tissue engineering to create biological wires that would seek out and communicate with the surrounding neurons.

In order to address the fork in the Jell-O problem, Martin suggested a number of changes that could be made to the electrodes that would make them less like a fork and more like another piece of Jell-O. In addition to electrodes that were "fuzzy" and had a greater surface area with which to interact with the surrounding neurons, he proposed creating a polymer or gel that approached the softness of the brain, but was still able to transmit electric current or to act as a scaffold for very thin electrodes.

But all of the potential attempts at bypassing the problem to make a better connection between the brain and the electrode boiled down to the fundamental issue articulated by Moxon, "We still don't know what it means to stick something in the brain." However, there was still disagreement as to whether the basic research should be completed before development went forward, or whether the two lines of research could progress in parallel.

At first those who primarily studied biological systems felt that understanding how brain tissue reacts should be addressed before one could think about designing a better electrode. To learn more about the problem itself, Kyriakides boldly stated, "I don't think the answer is going to come from the materials side," to the great frustration of group members like Martin, whose research focused on ways to engineer materials to make better electrodes.

After considerable discussion, it became clear that the future would require work on both fronts, and that work on one front could help inform work on the other. For example, the electrode itself could be used to study the effects of its own presence on the cells around it. Fashioning an electrode that could detect the chemical and cellular changes in its vicinity could inform biologists and provide a fascinating challenge for engineers.

Eventually, and beautifully reflecting the spirit of collaboration and the ultimate goal the conference itself, both sides began to see the usefulness of the others' approaches. "This is the first time I've sat in a room with people who talk like this," said Kyriakides. Many other group members echoed the sentiment. "This has turned into a much more productive session than I had hoped for," said Martin. By the end of the sessions the group members were discussing future collaborations. And the major hurdles in this field will require just this kind of team work.

Refine Technologies to Create Active Orthotic Devices

Background

Current orthoses were developed ultimately to enhance function of people disabled by injury to the limb (traumatic transaction of muscle and peripheral nerve) or by disorders that interfere with the muscle-nervous system, such as muscular dystrophies, stroke, spinal cord injuries, and weakness from aging. With few exceptions, currently marketed orthotic devices are passive and designed to overcome the weakness and instability produced by the pathology as well as to maintain the limb in an optimum functional position. The most common example is the polypropylene ankle-foot orthosis (AFO) designed to keep the foot and ankle at 90° to optimize foot contact and prevent foot drop in swing phase. The thermoplastic AFO is often designed with an articulating element between the foot and shank segments, thus allowing the patient some ankle motion. More elaborate braces for persons with spinal cord paralysis generally include the theromoplastic AFO linked to metallic uprights on the inner and outer shank and thigh. The uprights can even extend to a waist belt or trunk support (e.g., knee-ankle-foot orthosis [KAFO] or hip-KAFO. Hinges interposed at the knee and the hip are typically actuated manually or by cable systems. Patient-based research shows that the functional advantage of using these orthoses are difficult to measure. This may underlie the observation that while many children wear orthoses, during the transition to adults the orthoses are abandoned. The bulky stiff plastics, while providing support for the joint encompassed, interfere with body center of mass transition during walking. Furthermore, more elaborate braces, such as those spanning the hip to foot, are heavy so that energy requirements to move the brace are additive to the energy demands imposed by the disorder. Energy measures show wheelchair mobility to be more efficient than ambulation with current hip-KAFO systems.

On the other hand, considerable research has been devoted to development of exoskeletal devices that can be used to augment movement of military personnel in particular. Also, work has been done in the area of functional electrical stimulation and direct muscle stimulation to capitalize on the inherent efficiency of the existing human system and decrease bulk of the orthotics. Actuators include series elastic actuators already introduced in an orthosis to enhance knee extension and potentially allow stair climbing for persons with weakness. Fuel-power artificial muscles relying on electric and most recently chemical power sources are awaiting implementation in orthoses. Sensors in use today integrate muscle activity and foot contact forces and relay information from limb movements (potentiometers, accelerometers). Integration of the actuator and sensor technology requires computer algorithms to assure human movement stability. Motion laboratories are also required to appreciate the impact of the pathology and for testing the orthotic/exoskeletal devices.

Initial Challenges to Consider

- Adapt current lower extremity exoskeletal device for the elderly and persons with disability;
- Design a closed loop control system coupled to actuate an AFO at the "ideal" time of the gait cycle;
- Consider materials for orthotic fabrication that are light weight and durable; and
- Develop a model system to predict the effect of limb/joint actuation on stability of the person.

Initial References

Bakker, J. P., I. J. de Groot, H. Beckerman, B. A. de Jong, and G. J. Lankhorst. 2000. The effects of knee-ankle-foot orthoses in the treatment of Duchenne muscular dystrophy: Review of the literature. Clinical Rehabilitation 14(4):343-359.

Carlson, J. D., W. Matthis, and J. R. Toscano. 2001. Smart prosthetics based on magnetorheological fluid. Proceedings of SPIE 43:4332-4336.

Ebron, V. H., Z. Yang, D. J. Seyer, M. E. Kozlov, J. Oh, H. Xie, J. Razal, L. Hall, J. Ferraris, A. MacDiarmid, and R. Baughman. 2006. Fuel-powered artificial muscles. Science 311(5767):1580-1583.

Gard, S. A., and S. Fatone. 2004. Biomechanics of lower limb function and gait. ISPO Consensus Conference on "Orthotic Management of Stroke Patients," Ellecom, The Netherlands, September 21-26.

Guizzo, R., and H. Goldstein. 2005. The rise of the body bots. IEEE Spectrum 42(10): 50-56.

Kazerooni, H., R. Steger, and L. Huang. 2006. Hybrid control of the Berkeley lower extremity exoskeleton (BLEEX). International Journal of Robotic Research 25(5-6):561-573.

Lyons, G. M., T. Sinkjaer, J. H. Burridge, and D. J. Wilcox. 2002. A review of portable FES-based neural orthoses for the correction of drop foot. IEEE Transactions on Neural Systems & Rehabilitation Engineering 10(4):260-279.

Perry, J. 1992. *Gait Analysis: Normal and Pathological Function Intrathecal Baclofen for Generalized Dystonia*, 1st ed. Thorofare, N.J.: SLACK.

Pratt, J., B. Krupp, and C. Morse. 2002. Series elastic actuators for high fidelity force control. Industrial Root: An International Journal 29(3):234-241.

TASK GROUP SUMMARY

Summary written by:

Alla Katsnelson, Graduate Science Writing Student, University of California, Santa Cruz

Task group members:

• Mark Abel, Professor of Orthopedic Surgery and Pediatrics, Motor Analysis and Motor Performance Laboratory, University of Virginia
• Andrew Alleyne, Ralph and Catherine Fisher Professor of Engineering, Mechanical Science and Engineering, University of Illinos at Urbana-Champaign
• John L. Anderson, Provost and University Vice President, Case Western Reserve University
• Julia Chan, Associate Professor, Chemistry, Louisiana State University, Baton Rouge
• Kevin Granata, Associate Professor, Musculoskeletal Biomechanics Laboratory, Virginia Tech
• Andrew Hansen, Research Assistant Professor, Physical Medicine and Rehabilitation, Northwestern University

• Hugh Herr, Assistant Professor, Program in Media Arts and Sciences, Massachusetts Institute of Technology
• Zhiyu ("Jerry") Hu, Research Scientist, Life Sciences Division, Oak Ridge National Lab
• Star Hy, Booz Allen Hamilton, SETA Support for Program Manager, Defense Advanced Research Projects Agency
• Edwin K. Iversen, Vice President of Research and Development, Motion Control Inc.
• Alla Katsnelson, Graduate Science Writing Student, University of California, Santa Cruz
• Homayoon Kazerooni, Professor, Mechanical Engineering, University of California, Berkeley

Summary

Imagine two patients who present themselves to an esteemed rehabilitation specialist. One has a leg amputation, while the other walks with a severe limp.

On sight, diagnosing the first patient is easy—his problem would most likely be best addressed with a prosthesis to replace his absent leg. But diagnosing the second is another story. Is he limping because he's in pain? Or perhaps he lacks the ankle strength in his bad leg to propel it forward with the required force? Maybe his nervous system does not provide feedback to help him adjust his gait. Does he suffer from an injury that could get better or a degenerative condition that could get worse?

Despite the fact that twice as many people use orthotics as prosthetics, orthotics has remained something of a red-headed stepchild in the rehabilitation field. While recent innovations in adaptive or robotic approaches have potentially improved available prosthesis technology, these same technologies have not been applied to orthotic design, and clinical options for patients who could benefit from an orthosis have changed little in the last three decades.

The hypothetical patients above in part explain why. To some extent the goal of designing a prosthesis is straightforward—replace a missing limb. But for an orthosis each patient's condition defines the device's task. The disabled limb is a wildcard for an orthotist: Both its function and its deficits are unique to each individual. Conversely, many of the innovations that have revolutionized prosthetics (such as the C-leg and the rheo-knee) cannot be easily applied to orthotics, because there is no place to put them—if you already have a knee, albeit a bum one, adding another can weigh down the system. Much of the task group's discussion focused on resolving these difficulties.

Recently, researchers have begun to develop more active approaches. For example, Hugh Herr, head of the Biomechatronics Laboratory at the Massachusetts Institute of Technology's Media Lab and one of the task group members, is working on an adaptive ankle-foot orthosis. The device is able to adjust joint impedance based on the specific characteristics of an individual's gait. Exoskeleton systems such as BLEEX, developed by Homayoon Kazerooni, a mechanical engineer at the University of California, Berkeley, and a member of the task group, may also be used in an orthotic capacity.

However, most innovations have remained in the research realm, and are as many as 20 years from commercialization. The task group looked at ways to bring about an improvement over available technology within five years.

What's So Smart About That?

The first order of business in the task group was to define how active an orthotic could and should be. The team broke down the possibilities into three categories:

1. A completely passive device, such as those currently available, that could contain devices like springs that can store and release energy.

2. A quasi-passive orthosis that would contain elements that have actively controlled passive properties (e.g., controllable variable stiffness and damping).

3. A fully active system in which an actuator, such as a motor or engine, would generate force to augment or modify the patient's musculoskeletal movement. In the extreme case the system could control all of the movement and the patient would be carried along. The energy in this category comes from external storage, such as batteries or fuel. An exoskeleton would fall into this category.

A practical system may consist of a combination of the three categories. Because actuator technology remains heavy and weak, the energy storage concepts of categories 1 and 2 may provide insight into more efficient methods to accomplish category 3. Category 2 in particular requires an elegance and economy of design. Indeed, noted Herr, much of the difficulty lay in design: A powerful arrangement of springs, dampers, and perhaps small motors would store energy generated in the part of the movement a patient can make, to then be used in the stage where a patient's weakness lies. "It's like a hybrid car," he said.

The Taxonomy of Motor Control

As the discussion progressed, group members groped for a dose of practicality. Indeed, about half of the group had no experience with people who might use orthoses in their daily lives. Kazerooni noted that his lack of clinical awareness prevented him from seeing how to adapt his lab's exoskeleton to help people with disabilities. Other approaches, too, should be designed to solve a specific clinical problem, he said: "I'm trying to avoid developing a screwdriver and then looking for a screw."

Mark Abel, an orthopedic surgeon at the University of Virginia, showed a series of videos demonstrating movement deficits of children from his practice. In one, a boy with muscular dystrophy teetered forward on his weak legs unassisted. In another, a girl with arthrogryposis walked slowly with a cumbersome brace (reciprocating gait orthosis) on her lower body. The steel brace, said Abel, was the best technology could do, and yet she'd use less oxygen without the brace swinging her legs through with crutches alone. In many cases, he noted, it's the parents who want their kids to use the devices, because they approximate normal walking. Because they are so impractical, the kids themselves abandon their use by the time they hit their teens. "This little girl, if she doesn't walk by 12, she's always going to be in a wheelchair," Abel said, which in turn creates further lifelong health problems.

Based on the videos the group tried several ways to break down the problem. By disease was impractical; too many options. By a patient's degree of movement was inadequate, since the reason for a patient's impaired motor abilities would have to be key to the design. Finally, to loosely generalize the biomechanical task an orthosis would have to perform, the group decided on a mapping along two axes: neural control and muscle strength. The biggest needs, and the ones easiest to address with available technology, lay in the middle of the graph, the group decided—in patients who retained at least some of both muscle strength and neural control. This population includes a wide range of conditions, such as spina bifida, muscular dystrophy and cerebral palsy, and impairments associated with aging.

The graph provided a way to break down the abilities a particular patient retained; for example, a child with spina bifida may have functioning hip flexor muscles, so a device could be designed to take advantage of that.

Prioritizing Knowledge Gaps

In the second session a group leader emerged; a professor of mechanical engineer at the University of Illinois, Urbana-Champlain, who studies control systems, Andrew Alleyne, advised that the problem should be approached using classical design principles. He instructed each group member to identify the most pressing problem as they saw it. Ultimately, the group concluded that the key to a useful system was to create a set of modular design principles in which a basic device would address a general pathology, and components could be mixed and matched to an individual patient's needs.

By the final session the seminar room was wallpapered with five giant white sticky-notes, one for each key area where the previous day's discussion had pinpointed a research gap.

The needs in each area were defined as follows:

1. Control—we need a better understanding of how to take the right inputs and create the right outputs for a particular person with a disability.
2. Actuators—these must be smaller, lighter, faster, and stronger.
3. Power systems—better energy efficiency and management.
4. Sensors—better sensors of human activity would improve communication between the device and its wearer.
5. Materials—stronger and lighter substances that perhaps even contain functional features like actuators and sensors.

Prioritizing the five categories proved challenging, largely because they are so closely intertwined. Controls, actuators, and power systems are highly linked. Most orthotics frames are made largely of steel; if a lighter material were available, more weight could go to other hardware, such as the power supply. Power-to-weight ratio is less of a problem if the device can carry its own weight (including power systems) so the patient is not weighed down with this technology. One approach is to "re-motize" the heaviest components, including power systems and actuators.

Vigorous debate focused on the need to harness advances achieved in other fields. Orthotics is a deeply underfunded area—one group member noted that just two graduate programs in prosthetics and orthotics exist. Yet some of the problems identified in the group as key for new technologies are already active areas of study in other fields. "Maybe we shouldn't focus on energy supply," said Andrew Hansen, a prosthetics researcher who studies ankle-foot biomechanics at Northwestern University. "There's a whole Department of Energy. We should focus on issues specific to orthotics."

On the other hand, without better actuators the field was stuck, said Edwin Iversen, vice president of research at a Utah prosthetics company Motion Control. Others also noted that progress wouldn't be made unless solutions were specifically tailored for use in orthotics. Julia Chan, a chemist at Louisiana State University, Baton Rouge, who designs metal and ceramic synthetic materials, noted that she could think of possibilities for orthotics, but she and her colleagues had simply never considered the problem as they were not aware of the issues related to the field.

Much of the team agreed that the top issue was that of control—creating an intelligent way to channel feedback from both the device and the wearer into regulating the movement. "How do you drive a car when you don't have a good driver?" asked Kazerooni pointedly. One crucial aspect of this, noted Kevin Granata, a biomechanics researcher at Virginia Tech in Blacksburg, is that too little is yet known about the mechanics of walking in able-bodied people to predict the signals such a controller should use. In a person with neuromuscular conditions, muscle recruitment and movements are often dysfunctional, so the movement patterns recorded from the patient cannot be used as a reliable reference to control a smart orthosis. Developing a reliable and active system for telling an actuator what to do would open up many possibilities. "We don't know what to send to the computer," Kazerooni summed up. "That's the area of research."

Structural Tissue Interfaces: Enabling and Enhancing Continual Maintenance and Adaptation to Mechanical and Biologic Factors

Background

Successful implantation of devices that employ a direct structural interface with native tissues and organs requires the development of an intimate and symbiotic relationship enabling effective transmission of both mechanical and biologic signals. Furthermore, these mechanical and biologic signals serve as important regulators of the structure and function of the interface tissues. As a result, long-term incorporation and maintenance of an effective structural tissue interface will depend on the delivery of "just the right" signals.

From a design optimization perspective, an approach to the development of robust tissue interfaces would include the fabrication of implants that mimic the structure, mechanical properties, and biologic behavior of native tissue. An alternative strategy might include the design of an implant with generic properties that can rapidly adapt to the local environment (mechanical and biologic) by remodeling its structure and material properties. Clearly, these strategies are interrelated and depend on the creation of local niches inducing normal behavior of cells, matrices, and bioregulatory factors.

Initial Challenges to Consider

• Despite the recognized need for the creation of optimized local mechanical conditions, the characteristics of mechanical signals required for tissue maintenance remain incompletely understood. What are the critical mechanical conditions that regulate cell behavior at the interface? What are the mechanisms that enable the transduction and response to these mechanical signals?

• Long-term maintenance of a structural tissue interface requires the creation of a biodynamic interaction between the implant surface and the native tissue. What are the morphologic, architectural, and biomaterial features that promote the creation of this biodynamic interface?

• The strategies to create lasting interfaces might include the use of engineered materials that are inert or degradeable and induce effective tissue ongrowth or replacement, or the use of biologically based biomaterials that become incorporated and inherently part of the native tissue composite. What are the critical design features and parameters that would enable long-term incorporation and function at the tissue interface?

Initial References

Bonadio, J., S. A. Goldstein, and R. J. Levy. 1998. Gene therapy for tissue repair and regeneration. Advanced Drug Delivery Reviews 33:53-69.

Grodzinsky, A. J., R. D. Kamm, and D. A. Lauffenberger. 1997. Quantitative aspects of tissue engineering: Basic issues in kinetics, transport and mechanics. In *Textbook of Tissue Engineering*, eds. R. Lanza, R. Langer, and W. Chick, pp. 193-207. Philadelphia: Landes.

Fyhrie, D. P., and D. R. Carter. 1986. A unifying principle relating stress to trabecular morphology. Journal of Orthopaedic Research 4:304-317.

Huiskes, R., H. Weinans, H. J. Grootenboer, M. Dalstra, B. Fudala, and T. J. Slooff. 1987. Adaptive bone-remodeling theory applied to prosthetic-design analysis. Journal of Biomechanics 20(11/12):1135-1150.

Ingber, D. 1991. Integrins as mechanochemical transducers. Current Opinion in Cell Biology 3:841-848.

TASK GROUP SUMMARY

Summary written by:

Karen Schrock, Science, Health, and Environmental Reporting Program, New York University

Task group members:

- William Bunney Jr., Distinguished Professor; Della Martin Chair of Psychiatry, Department of Psychiatry and Human Behavior, University of California, Irvine
- Karen Burg, Hunter Endowed Chair and Professor, Bioengineering Department, Clemson University
- Steve Goldstein, Henry Ruppenthal Professor, Orthopaedic Surgery and Bioengineering Department, University of Michigan
- Danielle Kerkovich, Ph.D., Rehabilitation Research and Development Service, Department of Veterans Affairs
- Challa Kumar, Group Leader, Nanofabrication, Center for Advanced Microstructures and Devices, Louisiana State University
- Naomi Murray, Senior Research Engineer, R&D Technology Development, Stryker Orthopaedics
- Maria Pellegrini, Vice President for Research, Brandeis University
- Walter Racette, Director, Certified Prosthetist/Orthotist, Assistant Clinical Professor, Department of Orthopaedic Surgery, University of California, San Francisco
- Robert Sah, Professor and Vice Chair, Department of Bioengineering, University of California, San Diego
- Karen Schrock, Science, Health, and Environmental Reporting Program, New York University
- Dustin Tyler, Assistant Professor, Biomedical Engineering, Case Western Reserve University

Summary

Every prosthetic device—whether inside or outside the body, permanent or temporary, and regardless of the material it is made out of—will at some point abut the body's native tissue. This interface, in order to be smart, must enable the device to work with the body in order to allow the prosthetic to function as a living part of the system.

At the Keck *Futures Initiative* Conference in November, task group 6 faced the challenge of defining the characteristics of such a smart structural interface and identifying the gaps in current knowledge and technology that must be closed before a smart interface can be achieved.

The first order of business was to define the problem. Everyone agreed that a smart interface needs to be adaptable within the body's changing milieu, and capable of remodeling so that it does not degrade and can continue to adapt. The interface also must be stable and able to withstand different stresses and situations. But these descriptions seemed too vague, so the group finally settled on a more specific statement:

> The challenge is to develop a durable structural interface with native tissues and organs that promotes a seamless and interdependent relationship enabling effective transmission of mechanical and biologic factors and signals.

The group identified the three key characteristics a smart interface must have as durability, seamlessness, and interdependence with surrounding tissues. A **durable** interface was defined as stable, functioning continuously for the lifetime of the prosthesis's purpose (e.g., as long as its user is alive for a permanent implant, or until the purpose of the prosthesis has been served).

A **seamless** interface, as envisioned by group 6, would enable a natural transition between the prosthetic device and the body's native tissue. This transition would most likely require a mechanical and/or biological gradient and be able to withstand different functional stresses at different size scales. The seamless interface connects a prosthesis to the body naturally from a cellular level through a macroscopic scale. In other words, there is no boundary (encapsulation) tissue separating the implant from native tissue.

And finally, a smart structural interface must be **interdependent** with the tissues surrounding it. The interface must be able to adapt to the ever-changing environment of the body—remodeling, self-healing, and growing, if necessary. This interdependent interface must also allow the prosthesis to communicate with the body and use the body's resources—a concept the group called "biopermissive." A biopermissive interface would allow bidirectional biological signaling (mechanical, chemical, and electrical), and it would use the body's nutrients, resources, and waste disposal mechanisms (for both metabolic and wear waste).

In order to illustrate these abstract ideas, the group chose a model system for which to design an intelligent interface: an osseointegrated prosthetic limb that joins with the bone, muscle, tendons, and nerves in the body, and protrudes through the skin. The three essential characteristics—durability, seamlessness, and interdependence—present unique challenges when discussing bone, muscle, nerve, etc.

Durability for all the individual interfaces (skin, bone, and nerve) means that the prosthetic interface must be stable and robust, lasting for the lifetime of the user. In the case of the nerve interface, "durable" must include stable signaling that does not change over time.

Seamlessness and interdependence, however, are related to one another and require a more complex description. Skin, bone, and nerve interfaces in the osseointegrated prosthetic limb require different considerations. For skin a seamless interface must allow both a mechanical and biological gradient to exist, so that the skin will adhere to the protruding prosthesis even through subtle movements, and so that the skin will grow with it, treating it as part of the body, and allowing signals to pass between the prosthesis and native tissue. An analog system already exists in fingernails, the tooth-gum interface, and horns and tusks in animals. The challenge is to understand the signaling that happens at these natural interfaces so that it can be replicated in an artificial interface, thus enabling interdependence between the skin and the prosthesis. A truly seamless, interdependent interface at the skin would control infection, allow re-epithelization of the skin and remodeling of the prosthesis by taking advantage of nutrients in the body, and perhaps even enable vascularization of the prosthesis.

The bone interface also must have a mechanical gradient, able to evenly distribute stresses. In order to be seamless and interdependent, bone tissue must be integrated into the device (osseointegration), much in the way that bone remodels itself in the presence of orthopedic implants like artificial hips. In order for this to be a successful integration, the geometry and topology of the surface must be designed to work with the body and have a smooth mechanical gradient at many different size scales. The biopermissive interface must also enable remodeling of both the bone and prosthesis, through biological signaling and interdependent use of synthetic and biologic resources.

A seamless and interdependent nerve interface is perhaps the biggest challenge in a smart osseointegrated prosthetic limb. Seamless and interdependence of the nerve interface are reflected in two aspects of the interface with the nervous system. The first aspect involves the local molecular signals and pathways that control the interface with the engineered system. In the most biomimetic system the nerves would form synaptic connections to the device. This requires several incompletely understood signals to form the connection and an even less understood continual set of signals to maintain the connection indefinitely. The device also needs to match the mechanical characteristics of the nerve. In the inflammation cascade the device should not promote a long-term fibrous capsule that separates the device from the nerves. The presence of the device cannot disrupt the ionic balance of the local environment, which could affect the function of the nerves. The second aspect of the neural interface is signaling from information flow. In the example of an osseointegrated prosthetic, the nerve interface needs to extract information from the electroactivity of the nerves to interpret user intention and it needs to produce artificial activity to communicate sensory information to the user. There are thousands of axons within a single peripheral nerve. Communicating individually with each of these fibers, routing this information to a processor to interpret the information, and sending information to the interface are all challenges to be addressed.

So how will scientists create these durable, seamless, and interdependent interfaces between prostheses and native tissues? The group identified the gaps in current knowledge and research tools to acquire the knowledge that must be closed before such an interface can be designed.

Most importantly, in order for an interface to allow a prosthesis to virtually become part of the body, we must understand the multitude of interdependent systems that exist within the body. This includes cellular signaling, nutrient delivery and waste disposal, immune response, and the nervous system, among others. Although we understand much about how these systems function normally or in the presence of foreign bodies, such as an implanted prosthesis, their relationships with one another in the presence of implantable prostheses remain poorly understood. In order to design an interface that will function as a part of the body, we need to understand how native systems interrelate and influence one another in the presence of said prosthesis.

A specific challenge within this systemic approach is understanding mechanotransduction. How do external stimuli impact cellular activity? Evidence suggests that mechanotransduction, heat, and other factors play a much greater role in gene and subsequent protein expression patterns than originally believed. In order to create a biopermissive interface that allows signaling for nutrient exchange, waste disposal, or immune response, we need to develop a greater understanding of all of the factors involved in gene expression and how those factors might influence one another in a multifactorial environment.

In order to acquire such knowledge certain technological hurdles must be overcome. Models must be developed that take into account multiple biological systems so that interfaces can be evaluated in a realistic environment, such as the 3-D liver system known as "liver on a chip." Developing in vitro assays, in vivo model systems, and computational or virtual analyses using high-resolution imaging techniques, metabolic imaging, and appropriate algorithms will do much to promote our understanding of structural interfaces between man and machine.

Once biologically relevant in vitro systems are developed, high-throughput testing methods will need to be employed. In this way many different structural interfaces can be tested in a variety of scenarios by nondestructive means.

Task group 6 concluded that in order to develop these technologies and acquire systems-level knowledge, collaboration across diverse fields will be necessary. Chemists, structural and molecular biologists, and macromolecular scientists will have to share their expertise in order to understand what will be required to create a truly biopermissive interface.

Even after the ideal interface has been successfully defined, technological hurdles remain to actually building a living system. The interface will have to utilize biological substrates and integrate biological and synthetic materials, such as proteins and synthetic by-products. The actual fabrication and assembly methods will have to be able to simultaneously handle different size scales from nano through macro, and incorporate varying moduli and porosity into the device and interface.

Although these hurdles are significant, if they are overcome, the benefit to society would be enormous. Based on the osseointegration model alone, there are myriad of new or improved applications for smart interfaces—in-dwelling catheters, feeding tubes, and joint replacements. When these and other challenges are faced, almost any prosthesis will become a living part of the body.

Sensory Restoration of Perception of Limb Movement and Contact

TASK GROUP DESCRIPTION

Background

Neural control of limb movement relies extensively upon the interactions between sensory feedback and motor activation in order to execute functional movement. Sensory receptors are pervasive, and are located in muscles, joints, and skin. These receptors supply information regarding muscle force, length and velocity of movement, joint position, and skin sensation, such as touch, pressure, and temperature. Various forms of paralysis interrupt the motor and sensory tracts, causing not only loss of movement but also loss of perception. Clearly, a sensory loss also occurs with limb loss due to amputation.

A smart prosthetic might be expected to restore both motor and sensory function, giving the user the ability to both perceive limb position and contact, but also integrating this subconscious information into the actual control of the prosthesis (or neural prosthesis). Current limb prostheses and neural prostheses have initially focused on the motor elements, either through the powered component of the prosthetic or the electrically stimulated muscles, or the control aspects, for example via myoelectric control or physical movement that is sensed. However, there is considerably less attention paid to the sensory aspects. To restore complex functions will require delineation of the specific information that is required, determining how

61

such information will be acquired, and determining how it will be utilized both in providing internal feedback in the control of the prosthesis and in providing perception to the user.

Initial Challenges to Consider

• What kind of information should be acquired in order to provide enhanced performance of the smart prosthetic? Smart prosthetics for various levels of dysfunction might require different degrees of feedback, and upper extremity applications might be considerably different than those in the lower extremity. What sensory information is necessary and sufficient for each clinical application?

• How do different prosthetic systems alter the type of information that is required? For example, are there fundamentally different control needs in an artificial limb prosthesis (i.e., attached to the person directly) than an unattached neural prosthesis (i.e., a robotic limb) for restoration of movement?

• What are promising sources of the necessary sensory signals, and how might they be obtained? What technologies will be required to acquire these signals? What are the practical challenges in introducing this into a wearable prosthesis, and how will these challenges be met?

• What type of information will be most useful to the user in improving his/her performance in using the prosthetic/neural prosthetic? How little information will the user require?

• How will sensory information be provided to the user, and how will he/she not be overtaxed by interpretation of the information to provide true sensory-motor integration in the control functions?

Initial References

Abboudi, R., C. Glass, N. A. Newby, and W. Craelius. 1999. A biomimetic controller for a dexterous hand. IEEE Transactions on Rehabilitation Engineering 7:121-129.

Riso, R. R., A. R. Ignagni, and M. W. Keith. 1991. Cognitive feedback for use with FES upper extremity neuroprostheses. IEEE Transactions on Biomedical Engineering 38: 29-38.

Sabolich, J. A., and G. M. Ortega. 1994. Sense of feel for lower-limb amputees: A phase-one study. Journal of Orthotics and Prosthetics 6(2):36-41.

Scott, R. N., R. H. Brittain, R. R. Caldwell, A. B. Cameron, and V. A. Dunfield. 1980. Sensory-feed back system compatible with myoelectric control. Medical and Biological Engineering and Computing 18:65-69.

Shannon, G. F. 1979. A myoelectrically controlled prosthesis with sensory feedback. Medical and Biological Engineering and Computing 17:73-80.

Sinkjaer, T., M. Haugland, A. Inmann, M. Hansen, and K. D. Nielsen. 2003. Biopotentials as command and feedback signals in functional electrical stimulation systems. Medical Engineering & Physics 25(1):29-40.

Van Doren, C. L., R. R. Riso, and K. Milchus. 1991. Sensory feedback for enhancing upper-extremity neuromuscular prostheses. Journal of Neurological Rehabilitation 5:63-74.

TASK GROUP SUMMARY

Summary written by:

Tom Zimmerman, Graduate Student, Grady College of Journalism and Mass Communication, University of Georgia

Task group members:

- Eric Altschuler, Instructor, Physical Medicine and Rehabilitation, University of Medicine and Dentistry of New Jersey
- Gary Berke, President, American Academy of Orthotists and Prosthetists
- Daofen Chen, Program Director, Systems and Cognitive Neuroscience, National Institute of Neurological Disorders and Stroke
- Joseph Francis, Assistant Professor, Physiology and Pharmacology, State University of New York Downstate Medical Center
- Brian Hafner, Research Director, Prosthetics Research Study
- Stuart Harshbarger, System Integrator, The Applied Physics Laboratory, Johns Hopkins University
- Jack Kotovsky, Engineer, Meso Micro and NanoTechnology, Lawrence Livermore National Laboratory
- Cato Laurencin, University Professor, Department of Orthopedic Surgery, University of Virginia Health System
- Gerald Loeb, Professor, Biomedical Engineering, University of Southern California
- Mahesh Mohanty, Project Manager, Advanced Technology, Stryker Orthopaedics
- Marcia O'Malley, Assistant Professor, Mechanical Engineering and Materials Science, Rice University
- Steve Potter, Assistant Professor, Laboratory for Neuroengineering, Georgia Institute of Technology

• Joseph Schulman, President and Chief Scientist, Alfred Mann Foundation
• Dennis Turner, Professor of Neurosurgery, Neurobiology, and Neuroengineering, Duke University Medical Center
• Tom Zimmerman, Graduate Student, Grady College of Journalism and Mass Communication, University of Georgia

Summary

The loss of a limb and all its functions is the devastating and inevitable first consequence of amputation. In recent decades, however, science, medicine, and technology have become increasingly good at crudely replacing the physical limb itself. And while a new prosthetic hand and arm make it possible to pick up a cup of coffee, what's missing is the sense of where the artificial limb is in relation to the body, whether the cup is hot or not, and whether one's grip is coming perilously close to slipping or shattering the cup.

Our group was charged with identifying ways that prosthetic devices might be improved, particularly in restoring sensations that were once generated by signals transmitted from sensory receptors in muscles, joints, and skin. If such perceptions could be mimicked and coupled with systems for controlling movement, it would be possible to create prostheses that deserve to be called "smart."

Our task group brought diverse talents to bear on this challenge, as it included experts on physical rehabilitation, neuroscience, physics, orthopedics, biomedical engineering, mechanical engineering, and materials science—to name only some of the disciplines represented.

On the first day, hours of spirited discussion yielded a concise statement of the group's task: "designing/developing/implementing a prosthetic/robotic limb with a sufficient level of sensory restoration/feedback to achieve functional manual control." The group defined sensation broadly, including all "somesthetic" modalities, such as vibration, posture, movement, touch, and temperature sensing. This sensory feedback should provide input for restoring manual control, which will be considered successful and fully functional when sensation, motor control, and perception are integrated.

Although there are many types of amputations and catastrophic injuries that disrupt sensation, the group decided to focus on three groups of patients needing upper extremity restoration: amputees who need replacement limbs, stroke patients and others who need exoskeleton structures to restore lost sensory and motor function, and those who need augmentation of function, such as an industrial application.

With these types of upper extremity problems in mind, the group drew a time line for developing new sensory restoration technology. The group identified three milestones on the path to their ultimate goal: creating systems that are better than current prosthetics, as good as normal limbs, and, finally, even better than unaugmented normal limbs. Users should experience an increase in functionality rather than perceived complexity over time; as Antoine de St. Exupery wrote in 1940, "Technology progresses from primitive to complex to simple."

Armed with a definition of the problem and milestones for development, the group laid out a structure for its solution. The status of research was summarized in three vital areas: sensory acquisition, sensory perception/feedback, and control. Within each the members of the group focused on identifying current technologies that will enable near-term goals, the evolutionary path of prosthetics, and areas of research that should be explored to reach long-term goals.

They began with strategies for acquiring peripheral sensory signals. Tactile sensors may be used to measure parameters of a contact between the prosthetic device and another object. These sensors may be biomimetic, capacitive, Micro-Electro-Mechanical Systems (MEMS), or quantum tunneling composites (QTC). Proprioceptive sensors, such as shaft encoders on the robotic limb or MEMS gyros and accelerometers, are essential for letting the brain know where the artificial limb is in relation to the body. Finally, there should be some means of communication, whether wired or wireless telemetry, to transmit sensory information to the system that controls movement of the prosthesis and to the operator.

Second, the group considered various strategies for presenting sensory information to the brain, either at the level of the central or the peripheral nervous system. Implantable electrode arrays were considered, but members were concerned that these might be mechanically unstable and might cause fibrosis. Targeted reinnervation was also discussed, but the group was divided about whether experimental surgeries were within the boundaries of the task we had set ourselves. The concept of sensory substitution was discussed, in which sensory data can be redirected from a damaged sensory site or modality to an intact one. There was some enthusiasm for the possibility that patients would obtain improved sensory feedback from residual sensation in the stump if the fixation of the prosthesis to the stump were improved (e.g., by mechanical integration into the bone).

Finally, different ways of controlling movement of the prosthesis were considered. One is a subconscious local control loop in the prosthesis itself, which is fast and reflexive but offers limited function and little perception. Putting the human directly in the loop, either instead of or in addition to the local loop, ought to make the prosthesis more adaptable, more easily customized, and thus more likely to be functional for patients and be accepted by them.

Having determined a structure for solving the task, the group turned to three gaps in current scientific knowledge and technology that need to be addressed. First, research is needed to learn which sensor technologies are best suited to prosthetic devices, which need cutaneous sensing of variations in pressure, temperature, and texture, as well as proprioceptive capacity. Group members agreed that there was a desire for implantable, low-power, high-bandwidth sensors that acquire simultaneous data in multiple modes.

A significant challenge is that providing conscious sensation is likely to feel invasive to users, depending on the type and location of the interface. If the sensory units are invasive, patients are more likely to accept them if they are also highly functional, long lasting, and reliable.

The second gap in scientific knowledge is that researchers are not certain as to ideal techniques to deliver sensory data from the prosthesis to the body to achieve optimal control of movement. Here the group was excited about numerous avenues of research. These included using sensory translation and sensory substitution to improve cutaneous representation. Intervention at the central nervous system level, such as brain implants with more sophisticated coding methods, is also of great interest. And whether the interface is in the brain or in the peripheral nervous system, mechanical interfacing that accommodates motion relative to the recording site is a challenge. As one group member stated, directly stimulating the central nervous system is like "throwing big boulders into the mainframe of a computer and trying to control it."

The group developed the idea of muscular proprioception, in which muscle power would be utilized mechanically and taking advantage of the built-in proprioception of muscles to provide feedback to the wearer. Further, the group realized the need for further psychophysical experiments to understand which types of feedback required conscious perception.

In terms of managing controls at all levels, the group posited utilization of the unimpaired limb as a controller as in teleoperation. Also, use of transmissions tied to muscles instead of relying on electromyography (EMG) signals would create better resolution. Finally, supraspinal interfaces for sensory input to the brain could be used, integrating it with existing methods for motor output from the brain. Group members then constructed a taxonomy of key control loops.

• Local smart—reflexive adjustment of the actuators in the prosthesis;
• Fast human loop—reflexive/spinal cord (brain is able to modulate the loop);
• Cerebral loop—for dexterous manipulation;
• Slow human loop—supervisory control, internal model adaptation; and
• Customization loop—based on user wearability, patient acceptance, training.

From this taxonomy the group identified several questions. First, what degree of local smarts is needed or beneficial to reduce computational and bandwidth load upstream? Second, how does one remain aware that they are grasping something in their hand via feedback? Also, how do you couple feed-forward and feedback control of prosthesis with adaptation to accommodate external system dynamics?

The group considered how much technology could be included in a prosthetic without making the device horribly complex and unfriendly to the user. First, the device must be easy to attach and align, especially for bilateral amputees. The interface and attachment materials will undoubtedly be very sensitive, which will lead to the potential for damage. The long-term stability of sensory input must also be examined. What cognitive demand will the smart prosthesis cause? Group members have debated just how smart is smart, and what is still required of the user? Finally, considering that many people have a low tolerance for learning to use their new VCR or cell phone to its fullest capacity, just how high will the tolerance be with this new "gadget"?

With all emerging technologies and scientific breakthroughs, there are certainly ethical and socioeconomic implications. Developing a smart prosthetic limb is no different. Who will fund the research and development of these new prostheses, particularly if the market size is small? As new technologies emerge, will they be available to all users, no matter their socioeconomic status? Will increased function require increasingly invasive in-terfaces, and will this lead to an increase in "designer surgeries?" Finally, if prosthetics one day do prove to be better than the average limb, will users with no medical need opt for voluntary amputation in order to seek in-creased function? Will the ability to interact telerobotically with a manipulandum that is remote from the operator provide desirable functionality?

The idea of a voluntary amputation is one that many group and audi-ence members found unnatural, but compelling for argument's sake. It is representative of a best-case scenario as defined by the group to allow a hypothetical teasing-out of ideas. This task group and the Keck *Futures Initiative* allowed experts from many disciplines to convene for eight hours of spirited discussion and occasional sparring, thinking big, and taking risks in solving a common problem. For now, however, attention will turn back to the first milestone on the timeline for solving the problem: constructing prosthetic devices that incorporate more sensory perception than those available at the present.

Design a Functional Tissue Prosthesis

TASK GROUP DESCRIPTION

Background

In recent years the approach to rebuilding tissues inside of the body or creating tissues outside of the body as in vitro models or for implantation has been focused on using tissue-engineering principles. Tissue building during development can be imitated by combining cells and/or biological factors with a biomaterial that acts as a scaffold for tissue development. Cells can synthesize new tissue as well as provide the signals needed for tissue formation. Biomaterials can be designed in forms that imitate the natural organization of the extracellular matrix. Signaling molecules can be bound or incorporated into the scaffolds to aid in morphogenesis, pattern formation, and cell differentiation. Currently, however, the quality and function of many tissue-engineered prostheses still need to be improved to fully address the clinical need. For example, skin can be replaced by the use of allogeneic keratinocytes and dermal fibroblasts on a collagen scaffold. This construct can form an epidermis, stratum corneum with barrier properties and a basal lamina in vivo. However, the secondary structures, such as hair follicles and sebaceous and sweat glands, do not develop. Many tissues have complex primary and secondary structures and functions. The goal is to design better tissue prostheses that mimic or model tissue.

Initial Challenges to Consider

Design a functional tissue prosthesis that effectively models the tissue being replaced. Select a tissue or organ that poses the greatest engineering challenges, such as neural tissue in the central nervous system, kidney, pancreas, and skin.

• Determine the desired characteristics/functions of the prosthetic device. Consider those features that have yet to be met by our current technology.
• Design a device that combines all of the desired characteristics you have identified.
• Consider cell type(s) and their source(s).
• Consider signaling molecules that may be mobilized, incorporated, and/or released in the construct.
• Consider the composition and design of the biomaterials acting as a template/scaffold.
• Consider instrumentation for improving interaction with the nervous system and/or brain.

Initial References

Anderson, D., J. Burdick, and R. Langer. 2004. Material science: Smart biomaterials. Science 305:1923-1924.
Bell, E. 2000. Tissue engineering in perspective. In *Principles of Tissue Engineering*, 2nd ed., eds. R. Lanza, R. Langer, and J. Vacanti. San Diego: Academic Press.
Griffith, L., and G. Naughton. 2002. Tissue engineering—current challenges and expanding opportunities. Science 295:1009-1014.
Hare, N., and S. Strittmatter. 2006. Can regenerating axons recapitulate developmental guidance during recovery from spinal cord injury. Nature Reviews Neuroscience 7: 603-616.

TASK GROUP SUMMARY

Summary written by:

Ewen Callaway, Graduate Science Writing Student, University of California, Santa Cruz

Task group members:

- Jennifer Byers, Recruiting Editor, Proceedings of the National Academy of Sciences
- Ewen Callaway, Graduate Science Writing Student, University of California, Santa Cruz
- Jennifer Elisseeff, Assistant Professor, Biomedical Engineering, Johns Hopkins University
- Boyd Evans, Research Staff, Biomedical Sciences, Oak Ridge National Laboratory
- Sarah Heilshorn, Assistant Professor, Materials Science and Engineering, Stanford University
- Joerg Lahann, Assistant Professor, Chemical Engineering and Biomedical Engineering, University of Michigan
- Treena Livingston Arinzeh, Assistant Professor, Biomedical Engineering, New Jersey Institute of Technology
- Seth Messinger, Assistant Professor, Sociology and Anthropology, University of Maryland, Baltimore County
- Roger Narayan, Associate Professor, Department of Biomedical Engineering, University of North Carolina
- Vilupanur Ravi, Professor, Chemical and Materials Engineering, California State Polytechnic University
- Jeffrey Schwartz, Professor, Chemistry, Princeton University
- Judith Stein, Chief Technologist, Chemical Nanotechnologies Lab Department, GE Global Research

Summary

No matter what we attempt to do, no matter to what fields we turn our efforts, we are dependent on power. We have to evolve means of obtaining energy from stores which are forever inexhaustible.

—Nicola Tesla

Sitting toward the front of the auditorium, we waited anxiously to tell an audience of more than 100 eminent doctors and scientists just what the group had been up to the past three days. While we waited, Boyd Evans, an engineer from Oak Ridge National Laboratory, compared the four-day event to a vacation. "It's like summer camp for scientists," he said with obvious delight. No merit badges were awarded, but the team's final presentation was a chance to prove its craftiness.

Minutes later several brave group members told the audience we had devised an organ, inspired by electric eels, we called the biological power pack. Borrowing a design similar to an eel's electricity-generating organ and using human cells, the tissue would generate hundreds of volts and could be used to power other electricity-hungry prosthetics and implants that were once the domain of science fiction: deep brain stimulators, artificial retina, and synthetic heart valves.

The group had presented an inkling of that idea a day earlier, and the plan was met with the skepticism that comes naturally to a crowd of researchers. "Now, how are you going to do that?" one audience member asked. A day later, after our final brainstorming session, we had a plan—or at least the shell of one.

The idea isn't as outlandish as it sounds. The crux of our strategy was to devise a way of translating the chemical energy that cells produce so expertly into a form more easily harnessed by machines. By using cells to generate that energy the organ instantly becomes more responsive to the whims of the human body. "Cells are the ultimate biosensor," said group member Sarah Heilshorn, a bioengineer at Stanford University.

Tasked with designing a functional tissue prosthetic, many in the eclectic group of a dozen weren't even sure what our assignment actually was. The team was heavy on materials scientists and bioengineers, a different cut from the neuroscientists and clinicians that made up most other task groups at the conference. But the group's diversity turned out to be one of its defining characteristics, said group member Jeff Schwarz, a chemist at Princeton University, who urged the team to think outside the box. "I tried to look for a topic that would be fun for everybody in that very, very heterogeneous group," he said after the conference.

Initially, the group was set on engineering a particular organ. "Once you can design a kidney, you can design anything," said Judith Stein, a chemist with General Electric's nanotechnology lab. Diabetes affects millions of people and is one of the leading causes of kidney failure. The current treatment, dialysis, is burdensome and often ineffective, so a replacement kidney would have a huge impact on people's lives, the group agreed. To come up with a way to design a replacement kidney, we decided to reduce the organ to its basic functions, including filtering the body's waste, maintaining blood pressure, and producing vitamin D and other hormones. If our team could address each function individually and integrate them later, we could come up with a complete working organ. A complication quickly arose: Integrating the myriad of functions any organ performs is easier said than done. We likened the task to an English faucet with separate spigots for hot and cold, where it's difficult to produce water at just the right temperature. By the same token, decoupling the functions of a kidney, or any organ, could make it difficult to integrate the parts.

With the artificial kidney scuttled, we looked to refocus our efforts. On the minds of many members was the theme of the conference—"smart" prosthetics. In a series of opening talks and tutorials, we had learned about devices like cochlear implants, spinal cord stimulators, and bionic legs. It dawned on the group that all the devices shared a need for power and lots of it. Batteries now power the prosthetics, but as implants become increasingly complex and more deeply embedded in the body, batteries become inconvenient and limiting. What if we designed a biological energy source that could run prosthetics independently, we asked. Such a power source could be customized to the needs of any prosthetic. "The more universal it's made, the better," said bioengineer Roger Narayan, from the University of North Carolina.

We ran with it. In a fit of creativity the group wondered how electric eels generate their trademark shock. A quick web search revealed the animals employ a series of specialized cells called electrocytes, able to generate up to 600 volts of electricity. The eel's electrocytes, which are half nerve cell, half muscle, are synchronized and aligned to maximize the electricity they put out. Nerve cells communicate with one another by creating a small electrical current that triggers the release of a chemical signal sent to neighboring cells. The eel cells perform that feat on a much grander scale. But the difference is like going from a string quartet to a 200-musician orchestra; the music may be the same, but the challenge is getting everybody to play together.

With time running short the team decided to break up into smaller groups to come up with solutions to creating the power pack, which we split into biological, material, and electrical. However, the team's goal was not to simplify the problem. "We don't want to find the easiest solution," said one team member. Instead, the group should "bring in as much complexity into the design as possible, so we end up with something novel that no one's thought of."

From a biological standpoint the idea's first stumbling block was its use of eel cells in a human body. To avoid an immune response the cells would have to be walled off from the rest of the body, making it difficult to supply the cells with oxygen and nutrients. The team's solution was to use human stem cells to create electrocyte-like cells that didn't provoke an immune response. Stem cells are pluripotent, meaning they can turn into other types of cells, given the right chemical cues. The plan was to first direct stem cells to become muscle, and then chemically divert them down the path to nerve cell. This would be a major challenge, said Jenifer Elisseeff, a bioengineer at Johns Hopkins University, but not an impossible one. In the last decade scientists have become increasingly adept at coaxing stem cells to morph into other types of tissue.

By studying the eel organ the group quickly discovered the arrangement of the cells was essential to the organ's function. The eel's electrocytes were arrayed head to tail to make electrical conduction possible. To re-create this configuration the group proposed using a microfabricated material with tiny built-in cups for each of the cells. The material could be coated with chemicals that promote cell adherence and correct orientation.

The final, and perhaps most complex, aspect of our biological power pack was the electrical power itself. Here the group consulted Gary Fedder, an electrical engineer from Carnegie Mellon University. He said the idea was feasible, but that it would have to overcome several technical hurdles. To generate an electrical current the cells pump charged ions in and out of their cytoplasm. The resulting electrolyte soup could dissipate any electricity the cells produce. Fedder also said the system would have to be designed in such a way that only the first and last cells in the series make contact with the electrical circuitry. Thus, the cells needed to be insulated, adding another layer of complexity to the design.

To jump-start the organ into action the team proposed employing a piezoelectric device, which uses crystals to capture energy from the body's movement. Once started the system would run on glucose, the body's own supply of energy.

With these considerations accounted for the group took the idea to the other conference attendees. At a scientific talk the best way to gauge interest is by the number of questions audience members ask afterward—the more, the better. By that standard ours was a resounding success, as the moderator had to cut off questions to allow time for other task groups to present. Many of the questions were skeptical, but none brushed aside the idea as quackery.

"Realistic is a time frame," said Jeff Schwarz, after the conference. "People are going to figure out how to harness metabolism and transduce it into electricity in your lifetime," he told me. A month after the meeting the group reconvened in a teleconference to discuss the project's next steps. The group plans to apply for a small seed grant from the Keck Foundation to fund a meeting to hash out more concrete ideas and perhaps a larger grant proposal.

"The final concept will likely be different from the group's presentation at the conference," said Vilupanur Ravi, a materials engineer from California State Polytechnic University in Pomona. But he said the task group meetings allowed the group to come together in a way that makes future collaboration easier, no matter the focus. The conference "can be an inflection point if our idea takes off," he said.

Create Hybrid Prostheses That Exploit Activity-Dependent Processes

TASK GROUP DESCRIPTION

Background

It is clear that a number of cellular processes within the nervous system are linked strongly to electrical activity within nerve cells. These processes include gene expression (West et al., 2002) and neuronal growth (Salimi and Martin, 2004), and patterned neuronal activity is also critical to neuronal cell birth (Diesseroth et al., 2004) and survival (Salthun-Lassalle et al., 2004). The link between neuronal activity and these activity-dependent processes may be through the magnitude and time course of intracellular calcium concentrations and subsequent activation of second-messenger pathways, as well as the dependence of release of neural signaling molecules on the pattern of neural activity. The release of neurotrophins (Lessmann et al., 2003), which contribute to neuronal plasticity and growth, is strongly linked to neuronal activity (Balkowiec and Katz, 2002).

In parallel with these scientific discoveries, engineers have developed methods to interface with and thereby control the electrical activity within populations of neurons. Fully implantable devices are available to stimulate reliably neurons in the brain, within the spinal cord, and in the peripheral nervous system. Electrical stimulation provides the ability to control electrical activity within neurons and therefore provides a means to enhance and control these activity-dependent processes.

Initial Challenges to Consider

Therefore, it should be feasible to bring together science and engineering to create hybrid prosthetic devices that employ regulated patterns of neuronal activity to harness the activity-dependent processes in neurons. In contrast to current implementations electrical stimulation of the nervous system as a modality to restore function (Peckham and Knutson, 2005), electrical stimulation becomes a modality to augment regeneration, repair, and plasticity in the nervous system (Grill et al., 2001). The prosthesis is the means to an end rather than the end itself.

This task group will examine the potential of and challenges associated with the use of electrical activation of the nervous system to provide a means to regulate activity-dependent biological processes in the nervous system, and thereby to create a hybrid prosthesis to exploit these processes.

Initial References

Balkowiec, A., and D. M. Katz. 2002. Cellular mechanisms of activity-dependent release of native BDNF from hippocampal neurons. Journal of Neuroscience 22:10399-10407.

Deisseroth, K., S. Singla, H. Toda, M. Monje, T. D. Palmer, and R. C. Malenka. 2004. Excitation-neurogenesis coupling in adult neural stem/progenitor cells. Neuron 42: 535-552.

Grill, W. M., J. W. McDonald, W. H. Heetderks, J. D. Kocsis, M. Weinrich, and P. H. Peckham. 2001. At the interface: Convergence of neural regeneration and neural prostheses for restoration of function. Journal of Rehabilitation Research and Development 38:633-639.

Lessmann, V., K. Gottmann, and M. Malcangio. 2003. Neurotrophin secretion: Current facts and future prospects. Progress in Neurobiology 69:341-374.

Peckham, P. H., and J. S. Knutson. 2005. Functional electrical stimulation for neuromuscular applications. Annual Review of Biomedical Engineering 7:327-360.

Salimi, I., and J. H. Martin. 2004. Rescuing transient corticospinal terminations and promoting growth with corticospinal stimulation in kittens. Journal of Neuroscience 24:4952-4961.

Salthun-Lassalle, B., E. C. Hirsch, J. Wolfart, M. Ruberg, and P. P. Michel. 2004. Rescue of mesencephalic dopaminergic neurons in culture by low-level stimulation of voltage-gated sodium channels. Journal of Neuroscience 24:5922-5930.

West, A. E., E. C. Griffith, and M. E. Greenberg. 2002. Regulation of transcription factors by neuronal activity. Nature Reviews Neuroscience 3:921-931.

TASK GROUP SUMMARY

Summary written by:

Erica Naone, Graduate Student, Science Writing, Massachusetts Institute of Technology

Task group members:

• Rory Cooper, Distinguished Professor, FISA/Paralyzed Veterans of America Chair, Rehabilitation Science and Technology, University of Pittsburgh
• Robert C. Froemke, Postdoc, Otolaryngology Department, University of California, San Francisco
• Warren M. Grill, Associate Professor, Biomedical Engineering and Surgery, Duke University
• Ranu Jung, Associate Professor of Bioengineering and Co-Director, Center for Adaptive Neural Systems, The Biodesign Institute, Arizona State University
• Cameron McIntyre, Assistant Professor, Biomedical Engineering, Cleveland Clinic
• Erica Naone, Graduate Student, Science Writing, Massachusetts Institute of Technology
• Sasha (Alexander) Rabchevsky, Assistant Professor, Physiology, Spinal Cord and Brain Injury Research Center, University of Kentucky
• Patricia Shewokis, Associate Professor and Movement Scientist, College of Nursing and Health Professions, Drexel University
• Michael E. Tompkins, President, Animated Prosthetics Inc.
• Michael Weinrich, Director, National Center for Medical Rehabilitation Research
• George Wittenberg, Assistant Professor, Neurology, University of Maryland, and Geriatrics Research, Education, and Clinical Center, Veterans Affairs Maryland Health Care System

Summary

Challenged to design a radically new type of prosthesis, the group members chose to target the needs of a stroke victim. Stroke is the leading cause of adult disability in the United States. More than 700,000 people in this country suffer strokes each year, and many are unable to recover the range of movement they enjoyed before the stroke. The group recognized a clear need for better treatments for stroke victims, especially treatments that could better address neurological symptoms.

When a person has a stroke that disables the motor system, therapies are available to help him recover function, so long as the damage is not too severe. Recent work has suggested that massed practice—focused, deliberate practice of a variety of tasks—can help restore function by building on the bit of mobility the person retains after the stroke. However, the group identified two problems with current therapies. First, in the case of moderate to severe motor disability, patients are taught to use their remaining function to take care of themselves rather than to recover the full function they knew before the stroke. For example, a writer who suffers this type of disability may recover the ability to feed himself but not the ability to type. Second, when the patient has no voluntary movement around a particular joint, there are no known restorative therapies.

If the person is too disabled to practice moving, therapists may be left struggling to find functional areas and abilities upon which to work. Unable to help him practice movements, they might wish to work directly with the motor circuitry of his brain. Here we have a problem of not knowing what is activated in the brain when the stroke victim tries to move. This lack of knowledge of the nervous system's internal state represents a serious impediment to designing a strategy that would bridge the gap between intention and action. The group realized this leads to the old, deep question of "knowing the internal state"—in other words, completely understanding the brain, a question unlikely to be solved in the near future. To avoid having to decode the entire brain, they recognized the need to identify the minimum amount of information about the internal state that might be sufficient for a useful prosthetic. The hope was to replace the current trial and error method of restoring function with a more focused approach based on knowledge of how neural processing is affected by brain lesions.

The prosthetic the group imagined would work differently from both traditional stroke therapies and other prosthetics. Where traditional stroke therapies might leave the patient dependent, this prosthetic would assist the patient not only with daily activity but also with fully recovering lost function, eventually making itself obsolete. Where traditional prosthetics try to replace missing parts, this prosthetic would serve to link existing parts, effectively connecting damaged brain and body to functional ability in order to restore independence.

To imagine the device clearly the group considered how it would address the *internal state*, how it would be *hybrid*, and how it would exploit activity-dependent processes to assist *plasticity*. With an outline for this device in place the group hoped similar techniques could be applied to facilitate the healing process for multiple types of neurological injury and disease.

Internal State

The group quickly realized that building this dream device and using it would require finding a way for the machine to interface with the human brain, spinal cord, and peripheral structures. The device would need to read the brain's signals and return signals that the brain could read and interpret. It would need to cooperate with and enhance the brain's ability to compensate and adapt to the environment and environmental challenges. Finally, it would need to prevent the patient's brain from forming potentially harmful adaptations in the process of recovering from the injury.

While the potential device might need to have a high degree of sophistication and bandwidth to interface with the brain's relevant processes, the group found examples of crude forms of that intimacy in current technology. One member described the integration he has seen between upper-extremity amputees and their prosthetic arms. Once people learn to use the arm consciously, he said, they begin to use it unconsciously, talking with their hands and gesturing casually.

This example gave the group hope that through the use of the cutting-edge technologies of today and the near future, it would be possible to build devices that link ever more closely to the humans they are meant to help.

Hybrid

The device the group imagined was hybrid in many ways. They imagined a prosthetic system that united the body's biological processes with the system's synthetic ones. The device could intervene on the body's behalf by applying electrical stimulation, activating engineered tissue, delivering gene therapy, or supporting and amplifying remaining mental or muscular function. At the same time it could record progress, receiving feedback from the body that would teach it which interventions were the most helpful and providing feedback to the brain that would fill in gaps left by neurological damage. Finally, the device would be a hybrid because it would serve a hybrid *purpose*. In one way it would work as a traditional prosthetic, assisting the body in carrying out necessary tasks. In another way it would be a prosthetic means to an end, helping to rehabilitate the body with the goal of reducing the body's need for the prosthetic's assistance.

To function as a means to an end the prosthesis would need to insert itself into existing circuits in the brain, so it could assist wounded neurological tissue. Since much of the brain's ability to control the body's systems and adapt to situations depends on neuronal activity, the prosthetic would stimulate that activity at the appropriate times or amplify the signals of a few intact neurons.

A hybrid prosthesis would be fundamentally different from a traditional prosthesis. Rather than allowing the device to remain in a static relationship to its user, the hybrid prosthesis would incorporate three elements: the user, the adaptable prosthetic device, and a training or therapeutic regime. In the course of the patient's use of the device these three elements would adjust in relation to each other so that the patient would be gradually trained to function without the device.

Plasticity

Plasticity is the ability of the brain to change in response to learning or experience. Devices such as the cochlear implant have shown the power of this phenomenon. While the cochlear implant has been very successful at restoring lost hearing, that success is not achieved by replacing the damaged cochlea with an exact replica. Instead, the device takes advantage of the brain's ability to reorganize itself to make good use of the auditory inputs the implant does provide. By harnessing the brain's inclination to adapt positively, a great deal of function can be restored in the face of hearing loss. Following this example group members hoped to make their device use the same helpful tendencies of the brain.

The mechanisms that control plasticity are activity-dependent processes; effects in the brain that have different consequences depending on whether the affected neurons have recently fired (see sidebar for more information). Group members intended the device to make use of these processes to increase positive brain plasticity at times when the patient is trying to learn to restore lost function.

Other suggestions for ways to increase the brain's receptivity to the device's interventions included inserting engineered tissue, stimulating the brain, and using rehabilitation techniques, such as focused, deliberate practice of a variety of tasks.

Questions and Recommended Research

While the concept of a new type of prosthesis seemed promising, the question of the internal state remained a major hurdle. The group tried to find ways to define the success of the device by measuring easily observable external signals. It would be necessary to know the internal state or some approximation of it in real time, in order to see what effect, positive or negative, an intervention was having.

The group's recommended areas of research and identified knowledge gaps focused on unlocking the mystery of these internal states and making use of them. They wanted to understand how plasticity works in an injured system, and to learn how to control, activate, and facilitate plasticity and recovery. The limits of plasticity also need to be discovered. Though much remains to be learned about the rules governing plasticity and its limits, the group agreed that taking advantage of the brain's plasticity mechanisms was desirable. To achieve that goal they suggested research into the following questions:

- How far is the brain able to adapt?
- Is there a limit to neuronal adaptation?
- Are there focal neural areas that need to be targeted for an intervention to be most effective?
- What are the critical factors, internal to the system, that enhance neural plasticity?

These questions are the beginning of the journey to solve the mystery of the brain, prosthesis, and function.

The connection of internal to external was also an area the group wanted to explore further. What would be an adequate way to represent the internal state in order for a device to interface with the neurological system? How could they drive a system toward a desired internal state and what might that desired state be? How could a feedback loop be set up between the brain and a prosthetic device?

In addition to addressing these questions group members also sug-

Activity-Dependent Processes: What Is Known
George Wittenberg

We know a great deal about the rules governing CNS neuronal plasticity in animal models. The most familiar model is LTP in the hippocampus,[1] in which coordinated pre- and postsynaptic activity leads to increased synaptic strength. LTP occurs at a synapse, at least partly, by a mechanism in which presynaptic release of glutamate onto postsynaptic NMDA receptors leads to an increase in synaptic efficacy, if the postsynaptic neuron is active close to the time of that release of glutamate. But there exist other mechanisms for LTP, with other important transmitters and mediators.

Besides LTP there are *homeostatic* mechanisms that tend to maintain mean neuronal firing rates near a criterion. One might not think that homeostatic mechanisms as supporting recovery, but if the nervous system were in homeostasis prior to injury, the firing rates of neurons would be changed by injury and homeostatic mechanisms might restore function by changing a few, more global parameters. Homeostatic mechanisms may be useful in development, may be detrimental after injury (e.g., by causing spasticity), and may underlie recovery from diaschisis. Homeostatic mechanisms include synaptic scaling, a nonspecific change in synaptic strength, and changes in neuronal excitability. Synaptic scaling is partly mediated by activity-dependent release of brain-derived neurotrophic factor (BDNF). BDNF is released and transferred to postsynaptic neurons in an activity-dependent manner.[2] Neurons regulate intrinsic excitability to promote stability in firing.[3,4]

There are also other synapse-level kinds of plasticity. Synaptic *augmentation*, a longer-lasting form of facilitation could enhance the ability of a neuronal circuit to sustain persistent activity after a transient stimulus, and this has been demonstrated in a competitive model of sensory integration in spinal cord neurons.[5] Long-term synaptic depression (LTD) is an important complementary phenomenon to LTP, because it can prevent runaway increases in synaptic strength and because it can reduce activity in ineffective neuronal pathways. Endogenous cannabinoids may mediate LTD,

gested more research into methods they hoped to incorporate in their hybrid prosthesis. For example, they suggested further research into the safety, efficacy, and reality of using gene therapy and tissue transplants. They also found promise in current approaches such as functional electrical stimulation and powered prostheses.

with the timing of their breakdown influencing the time window for long-term plasticity.[6] Endocannabinoids are important to glutamate-dependent motor plasticity in mice[7] and deletion of an endocannabinoid receptor is associated with reduced exploratory behavior. In summary, restoration of normal function in a damaged neuronal network depends on activity-dependent changes in excitability and synaptic strengths. Known activity-dependent mechanisms include synaptic scaling, changes in excitability, timing dependent mechanisms such as LTP and LTD, and shorter-term activity-dependent mechanisms such as synaptic augmentation. There are anterograde molecules—glutamate, BDNF, among others—and retrograde molecules such as endocannabinoids and nitric oxide. These processes and signaling molecules are targets for hybrid prosthetic interventions. Still, as Robert Froemke pointed out: Knowledge of how any of these factors influence actual neurorehabilitation in human patients is sorely lacking.

[1]Bliss, T. V. P., and G. L. Collingridge. 1993. A synaptic model of memory: longterm potentiation in hippocampus. Nature 361:31-39.

[2]Kohara, K., A. Kitamura, M. Morishima, and T. Tsumoto. 2001. Activity-dependent transfer of brain-derived neurotrophic factor to postsynaptic neurons. Science 291:2419-2423.

[3]Turrigiano, G., L. F. Abbott, and E. Marder. 1994. Activity-dependent changes in the intrinsic properties of cultured neurons. Science 264:974-977.

[4]Turrigiano, G. G., and S. B. Nelson. 2000. Hebb and homeostasis in neuronal plasticity. Current Opinion in Neurobiology 10:358-364.

[5]Nelson, P. G., R. D. Fields, C. Yu, and E. A. Neale. 1990. Mechanisms involved in activity-dependent synapse formation in mammalian central nervous system cell cultures. Journal of Neurobiology 21:138-156.

[6]Sjostrom, P. J., G. G. Turrigiano, and S. B. Nelson. 2001. Rate, timing, and cooperativity jointly determine cortical synaptic plasticity. Neuron 32:1149-1164.

[7]Gerdeman, G. L., J. Ronesi, and D. M. Lovinger. 2002. Postsynaptic endocannabinoid release is necessary for long-term depression in the striatum. Nature Neuroscience 5:446-451.

The Vision

If it is possible to extend current knowledge of the brain's processes to the necessary next level, people may be able to build the device the group imagined. One group member described what the device might look like for the person with the severe stroke.

The device he would wear would be a very "smart" hybrid prosthetic with many redundant systems. It would possess motors that could help move his limbs if necessary. It would be able to stimulate his muscles or his brain. It would be able to measure performance and adapt its function based on the measurements it made.

Maybe the stroke victim wants to reach for a glass of water. The system registers the initial signal from the brain that attempts to begin a movement in his arm. If he is successful and he reaches for the glass without any help from the device, it simply records the event. If, on the other hand, he is not able to do it alone, the device begins to assist, trying various strategies one after another. It would begin with the slightest interventions and if those were unsuccessful, would progress to the point that it used its motors (effectors) to move the man's arm for him if necessary. In the process it would observe which interventions worked and were most effective. Over time it could reduce the types of stimulation and intervention it used as the man recovered and gained better control of his arm. This long-term outcome would be considered analogous to skill learning of the very smart hybrid prosthetic.

The person suffering the debilitating neurological effects of a stroke represents one user who could benefit by exploiting activity-dependent processes to help the body help itself. But the work described above could be extended to improve neurorehabilitation for a variety of conditions. The more effectively the prosthetic can interface with the user, the more it could reach the seemingly unreachable cases that need the most assistance but are most difficult to help.

Can Brain Control Guide or Refine Limb Control?

TASK GROUP DESCRIPTION

Background

Decoding Brain Ensemble Signals

The possibility of brain control of artificial limbs became a realistic prospect when a population of brain signals recorded in the motor cortex of behaving monkeys was successfully decoded to provide accurate information about motor parameters (Humphrey et al., Science 170:758-762, 1970) and the direction of movement in space (Georgopoulos et al., Experimental Brain Research 7(Suppl.):327-336, 1983), even before the onset of movement. The first successful prediction of a complete, upcoming 3-D reaching movement trajectory was achieved shortly thereafter (Georgopoulos et al., Journal of Neuroscience 8:2928-2937, 1988).

Implanted Electrodes for Prosthetic Control

The application of this discovery for brain-controlled motor prostheses requires the chronic implantation of at least tens of recording microelectrodes inside the brain. To that end the main challenge in the 1980s and 1990s was to develop microelectrodes suitable for chronic implantation, such that they (a) would be made of material safe for the brain, (b) would maximize the number of recording sites per unit of electrode area (to limit the total number of implanted electrodes), and (c) would be associated with appropriate microelectronics to ensure signal amplification and pre-processing in close proximity to the recording site. Significant progress in all these three domains led during the past few years to a flurry of testing applications of neuroprosthetic control. Several laboratories are testing different kinds of systems of microelectrodes implanted in the motor and parietal cortices of monkeys and their capability for prosthetic control (for reviews see Taylor et al., 2002; Schwartz, 2004), and such applications on human subjects are also underway (Hochberg et al., 2006). However, major concerns remain. For example, the long-term (e.g., years) safety of implanted microelectrodes on the brain is essentially unknown, both with respect to the possible toxicity of the materials the electrodes are made of and the possible damage to the brain given the brain motion relative to the electrodes. However, the successful long-term safety and experience (>10 years) of much larger deep-brain-stimulating electrodes, used for the treatment of movement disorders, such as Parkinson's disease, suggests that the brain can tolerate at least some types of electrodes quite well. In addition, the length of time for which implanted electrodes will continue to provide good-quality signals for prosthetic control is also to be determined.

Noninvasive Brain Signals for Prosthetic Control

Ideally, it would be best to use brain signals recorded by noninvasive ways to control prosthetic devices. Substantial work has been done on using electroencephalographic (EEG) signals for the purpose of direct communication of the brain with the environment, for example, by moving a cursor on a computer screen. The use of EEG signals for prosthetic control would be a major advance and would bypass most of the safety and other concerns associated with implanted electrodes. In addition, since EEG reflects brain activity from many areas, such signals possess the potential of being useful in other applications, such as brain-aided cognitive therapy, rehabilitation, remediation, and biofeedback. Recent studies demonstrated the power of magnetoencephalographic (MEG) signals for predicting upcoming moment trajectories (Georgopoulos et al., 2005), using the same decoding methods as originally described (see above). Since MEG is noninvasive and complementary to EEG, these findings suggest that EEG would also be a good predictor, as indeed has been found in preliminary studies (Georgopoulos et al., 2005). Nevertheless, noninvasive studies cannot capture the single neuron scale of measurement as intracerebral micro-electrode arrays can, and the limits to such noninvasive information extraction have not been determined.

Initial Challenges to Consider

In the intact animal, signals from the motor cortex are directed to the spinal cord (from layer 5 pyramidal cells) as well as to other cortical and subcortical areas, all parts of a distributed dynamic motor control network. Ideally, the basic functionality of such a network should be incorporated in a prosthetic limb, in order for the full benefit and impact of using motor cortical signals to be achieved. This would be particularly useful for the simultaneous or temporally overlapping control of multiple aspects of limb motor function, including hand trajectory in space, opening, closing, or shaping of the hand, force intensity, etc. A first step in that direction might be to implement spinal-cord-like circuitry in the prosthetic limb (Georgopoulos et al., Science 237:301, 1987). The use of brain signals from multiple brain areas recorded from simultaneously (e.g., parietal cortex, cerebellum, basal ganglia) or extracted from noninvasive brain signals would provide integrating information from a wider network. Alternatively, such signals and/or network principles could be incorporated in the prosthetic limb. In other words, the drive would be for a "smart" prosthetic limb with a spinal-like circuitry and additional neural network integration inspired from known interactions among brain areas. The unifying point is to use the brain of the prosthetic to fill in the computation that the central nervous system naturally provides when motor intention is generated. It is very possible that such a smart prosthetic limb would be much more amenable for efficient and effective control by brain signals of various motor functions.

Initial References

Georgopoulos, A. P., F. J. Langheim, A. C. Leuthold, and A. N. Merkle. 2005. Magneto-encephalographic signals predict movement trajectory in space. Experimental Brain Research 167:132-135.

Hochberg, L. R., J. D. Serruya, G. M. Friehs, J. A. Mukand, M. Saleh, A. H. Caplan, A. Branner, D. Chen, R. D. Penn, and J. P. Donoghue. 2006. Neuronal ensemble control of prosthetic devices by a human with tetraplegia. Nature 442:164-171.

Schwartz, A. B. 2004. Cortical neural prosthetics. Annual Review of Neuroscience 27:487-507.

Taylor, D. M., T. Helms, I. Stephen, and A. B. Schwartz. 2002. Direct cortical control of 3D neuroprosthetic devices. Science 296:1829-1832.

TASK GROUP SUMMARY

Summary written by:

Kirk Fernandes, Graduate Student/Journalist, Center for Science and Medical Journalism, Boston University

Task group members:

- Richard Andersen, Professor, Biology, Caltech
- Jose Carmena, Assistant Professor, Electrical Engineering and Computer Sciences, University of California, Berkeley
- John Donoghue, Director, Brain Science Program, Neuroscience Department, Brown University
- Alexander Dromerick, Professor, Rehabilitation Medicine and Neurology Department, National Rehabilitation Hospital/Georgetown University
- Leon Esterowitz, Program Director, Bioengineering and Environmental Systems, National Science Foundation
- Kirk Fernandes, Graduate Student/Journalist, Center for Science and Medical Journalism, Boston University
- Apostolos Georgopoulos, Regents Professor, Director, The Domenici Research Center for Mental Illness Department, University of Minnesota Medical School
- Simon Giszter, Associate Professor, Neurobiology and Anatomy, Drexel University College of Medicine
- Selcuk Guceri, Dean, College of Engineering, Drexel University
- Jiping He, Professor and Director, Bioengineering and Center for Neural Interface Design, Arizona State University
- Leigh Hochberg, Instructor/Investigator, Neurology/Neuroscience Department, Harvard Medical School/Massachusetts General Hospital/ Brown University/VAMC
- Robert Kirsch, Associate Professor, Biomedical Engineering, Case Western Reserve University
- Zelma Kiss, Assistant Professor of Clinical Neurosciences, University of Calgary

• Conrad Kufta, Director of Clinical Development, Innovative Neurotronics Inc.
• Steven Schiff, Brush Chair Professor of Engineering, Center for Neural Engineering, The Pennsylvania State University
• Arthur M. Sherwood, Science and Technology Advisor, National Institute on Disability and Rehabilitation Research (NIDRR), U.S. Department of Education

Summary

It seems that in life the most effortless actions can be the most challenging to artificially replicate. Consider the simple task of picking up and drinking a cup of water. In the simplest terms that task starts with an intention to pick up the cup. The intention sets off movement-related neurons to "fire" or "spike" in our brains. Signals travel through the nervous system, leaping across synapses between neurons, activating the final common path of motorneurons, and eventually communicating with the actuators (muscles) of the limb. The arm, hand, and fingers move toward the cup. The visual system observes and reports progress, as do sensory neurons in our fingertips, hands, and arms report information, such as position and velocity, back to our brain, which then sends additional signals to adjust movement accordingly based on our expectations. Eventually the cup has made it to our mouth and we take a sip, invoking another set of complex but effortless functions. The key to making effective smart prosthetics may lie in understanding the complex interactions originating in our brains.

An assemblage of 15 scientists, doctors, and agency representatives with backgrounds ranging from neuroscience to engineering welcomed the challenge during the 2006 Keck *Futures Initiative* Conference by tackling the question: Can brain control guide or refine limb control? "Brain control" refers to the process by which information about desired limb movement is recorded directly from neurons in a patient's brain, decoded, and communicated to a smart prosthetic device that would then execute the desired movements. Following some discussion on the subject, the group submitted an answer to the query: "Yes"—as several participants have been involved in animal and human research that proves the basic concepts governing guidance via brain-machine interface. In moving ahead group members concentrated on the challenges of a brain-controlled smart prosthetic system, such as long-term stability, that when addressed, could advance the ability of the device to restore desired movement to a person with a physical disability.

In organizing the discussion one task group member suggested dividing the functionality of a brain-control system into three parts: command, communication, and control. **Command** refers to the implicit neuronal instructions generated by a patient's intention to move a limb. The brain-machine command interface records and decodes that data in such a way that the information is both manageable and useful for the desired movement goals of the system.

The **communication** scheme then relays the data to the prosthetic device through existing biological pathways or artificial mechanisms in cases of paralysis. There could also be a two-way stream of information transfer, as the overall smart prosthetic system might benefit from the ability to feed data back to the brain.

Control refers to the system that actuates the desired movement and ensures that the desired movement occurs regardless of disturbances—most likely a computer interface built into a prosthetic device that senses key variables and makes needed adjustments.

Due in large part to the range of expertise of the group's task members, the bulk of discussion focused on the command system. And in the end, participants took a holistic approach to addressing challenges, by creating a research roadmap for an ambitious goal-oriented initiative: develop a command interface that as a modular component in a smart prosthetic system, could fully restore function or have therapeutic value in the rehabilitation of lost movement.

The first issue task members needed to consider was the identification of the best targets in the brain for pertinent neuronal information. In other words, which specific neuronal signals, or combinations thereof, could be used to best determine the movement intent of the patient? Are the classical motor cortical areas ideal, or are the cognitive regions within the frontal and parietal cortices better sources for such information? The question sparked a lengthy debate over priorities when considering the most important variables of movement, such as trajectory, position, velocity, force, impedance, and posture. One participant noted that "pulling trajectories out of the brain is a piece of cake" and that velocity signals are "all over" in the motor cortex, but other variables were less studied. Other participants echoed concerns about a significant knowledge gap in this area, suggesting that it should be addressed in order to get a better handle on basic neurophysiology. They proposed a systematic research project that would study basic movements in healthy individuals to determine which variables were critical to specific actions and what corresponding neurons in the brain could be targeted for data retrieval. Additional research initiatives could prioritize motor requirements for restoration. Once the various patterns are fully understood, one group member suggested the possibility of developing a generator or model that could simulate key brain signals. Such a device would allow for easier experimentation with communication and control interfaces.

Once neuronal targets are identified, scientists then need to consider the best way(s) to record that information. Current systems use an array of electrical sensors to monitor neuronal action or local field potentials, but the methods vary in degrees of invasiveness. To date, the most detailed information with the largest signal-to-noise ratio comes from microelectrodes that are inserted directly into the brain via a surgical procedure. Some task group members noted there are still many challenges with this approach, including the long-term potential for biomechanical failure demonstrated through ongoing projects. In fact, one researcher questioned whether "this is the way to go," but another group member defended the method, saying, "There are many problems that remain to be resolved, but they are tractable." In any case, the task group suggested future research endeavors explore the creation of probes with built-in stabilization features that would automatically adjust to brain movement within the skull. Other issues to consider with such microelectrodes would be the need to fully implant the device (perhaps using wireless communication systems), redundancy, risk minimization, and Magnetic Resonance Imaging (MRI) compatibility. (Implants would ideally be designed for MR compatibility, as heating and tissue injury could occur otherwise; however, people with Deep Brain Stimulation (DBS) systems can receive MRIs following careful protocols.)

Continuing on the same topic, the group moved to discussion of the less invasive method of reading EEG (electroencephalographic) signals. While current EEG skullcap devices do not require the insertion of electronics directly into the brain, the signal-to-noise ratio is much lower in EEG recordings than microelectrodes, providing less valuable information, according to some task group members. However, at least one researcher was optimistic that with improved technology, an EEG command interface could be used to control limb movement or perhaps be integrated with microelectrodes into a network of sensors that achieve ultimate movement goals.

A secondary issue to consider when examining methods for *recording* is whether the same apparatus can also be used to *write* information to sensory neurons in order to provide feedback information to the brain. One scientist pointed out that some amputees request transparent prosthetic hands to ensure they have visual feedback on the proximal relationship between their hand and the object with which it's interacting. Such feedback would theoretically assist with adjusting and refining precise movements. One group member suggested that feedback signals could be processed in the prosthetic's control mechanism, then simplified before communicated back to the brain or peripheral nerves. Ideally through training, the patient could learn how to interpret these signals.

Once scientists have the pertinent neuronal targets and the optimal recording devices, they can set forth to optimize the decoding process with ideally quick algorithms that allow for rapid communication of brain signals to the smart prosthetic. The group did not focus on such decoding algorithms, but stressed the importance of adaptation in mechanical and computational systems due to potential neuronal aberrations in altered brains. An adaptive decoding system would learn as the patient's condition improves or worsens (in the case of ALS, for example). In addition, the group encouraged research that would support a co-adaptation strategy, in which both the command interface and control interface in the prosthetic would learn and refine movements together.

The group also put some attention toward considering the needs of disabled individuals when directing certain research initiatives. For example, one group member pointed out the fact that the great bulk of current brain-machine interface research focuses on arm movements despite the fact that the vast majority of amputation procedures are done on legs. And based on experiences with disabled individuals, other task group members stressed that ideal command, communication, and control systems should minimize attentional and training demands on the subject. Even public perception was a consideration, as the group wanted to dispel any general confusion over the phrase "brain control" and the false presumption that it describes a system that controls the brain rather than the prosthetic device.

Other issues that came under consideration included the appropriate representational frame for the prosthetic, the degrees of freedom required for commands extracted from the motor cortex, the required task effector, and whether movement specifications should be interpreted continuously, discretely, intermittently, or in some combination. Restoring complete

Preconference Tutorial Webcasts

**September 18, 2006, 1:00 p.m.-4:00 p.m. EDT
(10:00 a.m.-1:00 p.m. PDT)**

Closed Loop Systems to Facilitate Homeostatis

Robert F. Kirsch
Associate Professor of Biomedical Engineering
Associate Chair for Graduate Programs
Case Western Reserve University

Preclinical Trials, Translation to Humans, and Commercialization

Mark Humayun
Professor of Ophthalmology
Associate Director of Research
Doheny Retina Institute
Keck School of Medicine
University of Southern California

Medical Device Regulation: A Primer

Frances Richmond
Director, Regulatory Science Program
School of Pharmacy
University of Southern California

99

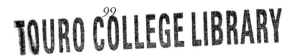

September 27, 2006, 1:00 p.m.-5:00 p.m. EDT (10:00 a.m.-2:00 p.m. PDT)

Prosthetics Applications in Plastic Brain / Learning and Training

Randolph J. Nudo
Director, Landon Center on Aging
Professor, Department of Molecular and Integrative Physiology
University of Kansas Medical Center

Engineering the Biointerface for Enhanced Bioelectrode and Biosensor Performance

Buddy D. Ratner
Director, University of Washington Engineered Biomaterials (UWEB)
Professor of Bioengineering and Chemical Engineering
University of Washington

Cell Instructive Polymers for Tissue Regeneration

David J. Mooney
Gordon McKay Professor of Bioengineering
Division of Engineering and Applied Sciences
Harvard University

Biophysics of Neural Stimulation and Recording

Warren M. Grill
Associate Professor of Biomedical Engineering
Associate Professor of Neurobiology
Associate Professor in Surgery
Department of Biomedical Engineering
Duke University

October 4, 2006, 1:00 p.m.-4:00 p.m. EDT (10:00 a.m.-1:00 p.m. PDT)

Neural Encoding and Decoding

Apostolos P. Georgopoulos
Regents Professor
McKnight Presidential Chair in Cognitive Neuroscience
Director, Center for Cognitive Sciences
American Legion Brain Sciences Chair
Professor of Neuroscience, Neurology, and Psychiatry
University of Minnesota Medical School
Director, Brain Sciences Center
Director, The Domenici Research Center for Mental Illness
Veterans Affairs Medical Center

Evidence for Aberrant Sensory and Motor Learning in Focal Dystonia: Implications for Learning Based Sensorimotor Training to Improve Motor Control and Cognition

Nancy Byl
Professor, Physical Therapy
University of California, San Francisco

Neural Biomaterial Interfaces in Tissue Engineering and Regenerative Medicine

Molly Shoichet
Professor and Director, Undergraduate Collaborative Bioengineering
Canada Research Chair in Tissue Engineering
University of Toronto

October 6, 2006, 1:00 p.m.-4:00 p.m. EDT
(10:00 a.m.-1:00 p.m. PDT)

Making Orthotics Smarter to Optimize Functional Ambulation for Persons with Disabilities

Bradford C. Bennett
Research Director
Motion Analysis and Motor Performance Laboratory
Assistant Professor of Research
Department of Orthopaedic Surgery
University of Virginia

Patient/Subject Risk Benefit Considerations from a Military Perspective

Kenneth C. Curley
Chief Scientist
U.S. Army Telemedicine and Advanced Technology Research Center
Associate Director for Science and Medicine, Center for Disaster and
Humanitarian Assistance Medicine
Assistant Professor of Military and Emergency Medicine, Surgery, and
Biomedical Informatics
Uniformed Services University of the Health Sciences

Patient/Subject Risk Benefit Considerations—Clinician/Scientist Perspective

Khaled J. Saleh
Associate Professor, Orthopaedic Surgery
Associate Professor, Health Evaluative Sciences Division
Division Head and Fellowship Director, Adult Reconstruction
University of Virginia

Agenda

Wednesday, November 8 (Hyatt Regency Newport Beach)

6:00 p.m.-10:00 p.m.   Welcome Reception / Registration, Patio Room

Thursday, November 9 (Arnold and Mabel Beckman Center)

7:15 a.m. and 7:45 a.m.   Bus pick-up from the Hyatt Regency Newport Beach to the Beckman Center
Van pick-up from the Island Hotel to the Beckman Center

7:30 a.m.   Registration (Outside Auditorium)

7:30 a.m.-8:30 a.m.   Breakfast (Dining Room)

8:30 a.m.-9:00 a.m.   *Welcome and Opening Remarks* (Auditorium)

9:00 a.m.-9:30 a.m.   *Keynote Address*
Michael M. Merzenich
Francis Sooy Professor of Otolaryngology
Keck Center for Integrative Neurosciences
University of California, San Francisco School of Medicine

9:30 a.m.-10:45 a.m.   *Panel Discussion* (Open Q&A with half the
                        tutorial speakers from the September and
                        October tutorial webcasts.)

Moderator: *Hunter Peckham*, Director, FES
Center, Veterans Affairs Medical Center,
Professor of Biomedical Engineering, Case
Western Reserve University

- *Apostolos P. Georgopoulos*, Regents Professor,
  McKnight Presidential Chair in Cognitive
  Neuroscience, Director, Center for
  Cognitive Sciences, American Legion Brain
  Sciences Chair, Professor of Neuroscience,
  Neurology, and Psychiatry, University of
  Minnesota Medical School, Director, Brain
  Sciences Center, Director, The Domenici
  Research Center for Mental Illness, Veterans
  Affairs Medical Center

- *Warren M. Grill*, Associate Professor of
  Biomedical Engineering, Associate Professor
  of Neurobiology, Associate Professor in
  Surgery, Department of Biomedical
  Engineering, Duke University

- *Robert F. Kirsch*, Associate Professor of
  Biomedical Engineering, Associate Chair for
  Graduate Programs, Case Western Reserve
  University

- *David J. Mooney*, Gordon McKay Professor
  of Bioengineering, Division of Engineering
  and Applied Sciences, Harvard University

- *Randolph J. Nudo*, Director, Landon Center
  on Aging, Professor, Department of
  Molecular and Integrative Physiology,
  University of Kansas Medical Center

- *Buddy D. Ratner*, Director, University of
  Washington Engineered Biomaterials
  (UWEB), Professor of Bioengineering and
  Chemical Engineering, University of
  Washington

- *Molly Shoichet*, Professor and Director, Undergraduate Collaborative Bioengineering, Canada Research Chair in Tissue Engineering, University of Toronto

10:45 a.m.-11:15 a.m.   Break (Atrium)

11:15 a.m.-12:30 p.m.   *Panel Discussion* (Open Q&A with the other half of the tutorial speakers from the September and October tutorial webcasts.)

Moderator: *Hunter Peckham*
- *Bradford C. Bennett*, Research Director, Motion Analysis and Motor Performance Laboratory, Assistant Professor of Research, Department of Orthopaedic Surgery, University of Virginia
- *Nancy Byl*, Professor, Physical Therapy, University of California, San Francisco
- *Kenneth C. Curley*, Chief Scientist, U.S. Army Telemedicine and Advanced Technology Research Center, Associate Director for Science and Medicine, Center for Disaster and Humanitarian Assistance Medicine, Assistant Professor of Military and Emergency Medicine, Surgery, and Biomedical Informatics, Uniformed Services University of the Health Sciences
- *Mark Humayun*, Professor of Ophthalmology, Associate Director of Research, Doheny Retina Institute, Keck School of Medicine, University of Southern California
- *Frances Richmond*, Director, Regulatory Science Program, School of Pharmacy, University of Southern California
- *Khaled J. Saleh*, Associate Professor, Orthopaedic Surgery, Associate Professor, Health Evaluative Sciences Division, Division Head and Fellowship Director, Adult Reconstruction, University of Virginia

12:30 p.m.-2:00 p.m.   Lunch (Dining Room) (Set up posters
                        throughout the Center)

2:00 p.m.-3:00 p.m.   *Perspectives on Neuroprosthetics from the View of*
                        a Neuroscientist and User
                        Alexander G. Rabchevsky
                        Assistant Professor of Physiology
                        University of Kentucky
                        Spinal Cord & Brain Injury Research Center

                        On the Design of Leg Prostheses: A Perspective
                        from an Engineer and User
                        Hugh Herr
                        Associate Professor of Media Arts and Sciences
                        NEC Career Development Professor of Media
                            Arts and Sciences
                        Massachusetts Institute of Technology

3:00 p.m.-3:15 p.m.   *Task Group Overview* (Auditorium)
                        Hunter Peckham, Chair, NAKFI Smart
                            Prosthetics Committee

3:15 p.m.-3:30 p.m.   Break (Palm Court 1 and Bay View 1)

3:30 p.m.-6:00 p.m.   *Task Group Session 1* (Locations throughout
                        Beckman Center)

Room	Task Group	
Crystal Cove	1	Replacing damaged cortical tissue.
Lido	2	Smart prosthetic to grow with a child.
Back Bay	3	Develop a prosthetic that can learn better or faster.
Irvine Cove	4A	Brain interfacing with materials.
Emerald Bay	4B	Brain interfacing with materials.
Palm Court 1	5	Create active orthotic devices.

Harbour	6	Structural tissue interfaces.
Laguna	7	Sensory restoration of perception of limb movement.
Bay View 2	8	Design a functional tissue prosthesis.
Balboa	9	Create hybrid prostheses.
Newport	10	Can brain control guide or refine limb control?

6:00 p.m.-7:00 p.m.   Reception/Networking

7:00 p.m.-9:00 p.m.   *Communication Awards Presentation and Dinner* (Atrium)

Honoring

- *Charles Mann*, author of *1491: New Revelations of the Americas Before Columbus* (Alfred A. Knopf), for his engaging and thought-provoking rediscovery of the early human history of our continent.

- *Elizabeth Kolbert*, staff writer, *The New Yorker*, for her authoritative treatment of the science and politics of global climate change in the three-part series "The Climate of Man."

- *Nic Young*, director, *Anna Thomson*, producer, and *Bill Locke*, executive producer, for The History Channel and Lion Television's "Ape to Man," an accurate and entertaining overview of human evolution made accessible to broad audiences. (Nic Young will accept the award on behalf of his colleagues.)

9:00 p.m.	Buses depart Beckman Center for Hyatt Regency Newport Beach
	Van departs Beckman Center for The Island Hotel
9:15 p.m.	Van departs the Island Hotel for Hyatt Regency Newport Beach (taxis will be arranged for the return trip)
9:00 p.m.-11:00 p.m.	Informal Discussions/Hospitality Room Hyatt Regency Newport Beach, Patio Room

Friday, November 10 (Beckman Center)

7:45 a.m. and 8:15 a.m.	Bus pick-up from the Hyatt Regency Newport Beach to the Beckman Center Van pick-up from the Island Hotel to the Beckman Center
8:00 a.m.-9:00 a.m.	Breakfast (Dining Room)
9:00 a.m.-11:00 a.m.	*Task Group Session 2* (Same meeting places as session 1) *(Beverages and snacks available in Atrium, Palm Court 1 and Bay View 1 from 10:30 a.m. to 12:30 p.m.)*
11:00 a.m.-12:30 p.m.	*Poster Session 1* 11:00 a.m.-11:45am: Session A posters are attended 11:45 a.m.-12:30pm: Session B posters are attended
12:30 p.m.-2:00 p.m.	Lunch
2:00 p.m.-3:30 p.m.	*Poster Session 2 (Beverages available in the Atrium)* 2:00 p.m.-2:45pm: Session C posters are attended 2:45 p.m.-3:30pm: Session D posters are attended

3:30 p.m.-5:00 p.m.	*Grant Program Overview* *Task Group Report-Outs* (Auditorium) (7 minutes per group including Q&A)
5:00 p.m.	Buses depart Beckman Center for Hyatt Regency Newport Beach Van departs Beckman Center for The Island Hotel

Evening on your own (a list of suggested activities is included in your conference packet)

5:30 p.m. and 5:45 p.m.	Buses depart Hyatt Regency Newport Beach for Laguna Beach
5:45 p.m.	Van departs the Island Hotel for Laguna Beach
8:30 p.m., 9:30 p.m. and 10:30 p.m.	Buses depart Laguna Beach drop-off site for both hotels
9:00 p.m.-11:00 p.m.	Informal Discussions/Hospitality Room Hyatt Regency Newport Beach, Patio Room

Saturday, November 11 (Beckman Center)

7:45 a.m. and 8:15 a.m.	Bus pick-up from the Hyatt Regency Newport Beach to the Beckman Center Van pick-up from the Island Hotel to the Beckman Center
8:00 a.m.-9:00 a.m.	Breakfast (Dining Room)
9:00 a.m.-12:00 p.m.	*Task Group Session 3* (Same meeting places as session 1) *(Beverages and snacks available in Atrium, Palm Court 1, and Bay View 1 from 10:00 a.m.- 11:30 a.m.)*
Noon-1:30 p.m.	Lunch (Take down posters)
1:30 p.m.-5:30 p.m.	*Working Group Report-Outs* (Auditorium) (20 minutes per group including Q&A) (Break from 3:30 p.m.-4:00 p.m. in Huntington Room)

5:30 p.m.-5:45 p.m.	*Chairman's Comments*
5:45 p.m.-6:45 p.m.	Closing Reception
6:45 p.m.-8:30 p.m.	Celebration Dinner (Atrium)
8:30 p.m.	Buses depart Beckman Center for Hyatt Regency Newport Beach Van departs Beckman Center for the Island Hotel
9:15 p.m.	Van departs the Island Hotel for Hyatt Regency Newport Beach (taxis will be arranged for the return trip)
9:00 p.m.-11:00 p.m.	Informal Discussions/Hospitality Room Hyatt Regency Newport Beach, Patio Room

Sunday, November 12
Leave for home. Safe travels!

SMART PROSTHETICS:
EXPLORING ASSISTIVE DEVICES FOR THE BODY AND MIND

Task Group Topics

Eleven interdisciplinary task groups will spend about eight hours developing a possible scientific plan to solve an outstanding challenge posed to the group. On Friday the task groups will give a short report-out (5 minutes each group) to share progress to date. A more extensive report-out will be completed on Saturday afternoon (about 20 minutes, including Q&A). The goals of the task groups are to spur new thinking, to have people from different disciplines interact, and to forge new scientific contacts across disciplines. The task groups are not expected to solve the particular problems posed to the group, but rather to come up with a consensus method of attack and a thoughtful list of what we know and don't know how to do, and what's needed to get there. The composition of the groups will be intentionally diverse to encourage the generation of new approaches by combining a range of different types of contributions. The groups include researchers from science, engineering, and medicine, as well as representatives from private and public funding agencies, university and business leadership, and science journals. Each task group will include a graduate student in a university science writing program. Based on the group interaction and the final briefings, the students will write a group summary, which will be reviewed by the group members. These summaries will describe the problem and outline the approach taken, including what research needs to be done to understand the fundamental science behind the challenge, the proposed plan for engineering the application, the reasoning that went into it, and the benefits to society of the problem solution.

Topics

1. Describe a framework for replacing damaged cortical tissue and fostering circuit integration to restore neurological function.
2. Build a prosthesis that will grow with a child (such as a heart valve or cerebral shunt, or a self-healing prosthesis).
3. Develop a smart prosthetic that can learn better and/or faster.
4. Brain interfacing with materials: Recording and stimulation electrodes. (Two groups will be run.)

5. Refine technologies to create active orthotic devices.

6. Structural tissue interfaces: Enabling and enhancing continual maintenance and adaptation to mechanical and biologic factors.

7. Restore sensory perception of limb movement and contact.

8. Design a functional tissue prosthesis.

9. Create hybrid prostheses that exploit activity-dependent processes.

10. Can brain control guide or refine limb control?

Participants

James Abbas
Co-Director
Center for Adaptive Neural
    Systems
The Biodesign Institute

Mark Abel
Professor of Orthopedic Surgery
    and Pediatrics
Motor Analysis and Motor
    Performance Laboratory
University of Virginia

Andrew Alleyne
Ralph and Catherine Fisher
    Professor of Engineering
Mechanical Science and
    Engineering
University of Illinois, Urbana-
    Champaign

Eric Altschuler
Instructor
Physical Medicine and
    Rehabilitation
University of Medicine and
    Dentistry of New Jersey

Farid Amirouche
CEO and President
Ortho Sensing Technologies

Richard Andersen
Professor
Biology
Caltech

John L. Anderson
Provost and University Vice
    President
Case Western Reserve University

Megan Atkinson
Senior Program Specialist
The National Academies
Keck *Futures Initiative*

Orlando Auciello
Materials Science Department
Argonne National Laboratory

Dennis Barbour
Assistant Professor
Biomedical Engineering
Washington University in St. Louis

Scott Beardsley
Assistant Professor
Biomedical Engineering
    Department
Marquette University

Ravi Bellamkonda
Professor
Biomedical Engineering
Georgia Institute of Technology

Bradford Bennett
Assistant Professor of Research
Research Director
Motion Analysis and Motor
    Performance Laboratory
Orthopaedic Surgery
University of Virginia

Theodore Berger
David Packard Professor of
    Engineering
Director, Center for Neural
    Engineering
University of Southern California

Gary Berke
President
American Academy of Orthotists
    and Prosthetists

William Bunney Jr.
Distinguished Professor
Della Martin Chair of Psychiatry
Department of Psychiatry and
    Human Behavior
University of California, Irvine

Karen Burg
Hunter Endowed Chair and
    Professor
Bioengineering Department
Clemson University

Jennifer Byers
Recruiting Editor
Proceedings of the National
    Academy of Sciences

Nancy Byl
Professor and Chair
Department of Physical Therapy
    and Rehabilitation Science
    Department
University of California, San
    Francisco

Ewen Callaway
Graduate Science Writing Student
University of California, Santa
    Cruz

Jose M. Carmena
Assistant Professor
Electrical Engineering and
    Computer Sciences
University of California, Berkeley

Julia Chan
Associate Professor
Chemistry
Louisiana State University, Baton
    Rouge

Megan Chao
Graduate Student in Broadcast
    Journalism
Annenberg School for
    Communication
University of Southern California

Daofen Chen
Program Director
Systems and Cognitive
    Neuroscience
National Institute of Neurological
    Disorders and Stroke

Ralph J. Cicerone
President
National Academy of Sciences

Jose Luis Contreras-Vidal
Associate Professor
Kinesiology, Bioengineering, and
    Neuroscience Program
University of Maryland

Rory Cooper
Distinguished Professor
FISA/PVA Chair
Department of Rehabilitation
    Science and Technology
University of Pittsburgh

Barbara Culliton
Journalist: Previously Deputy
    Editor, *Nature,* and News
    Editor, *Science.*

Kenneth C. Curley
Chief Scientist
U.S. Army Telemedicine and
    Advanced Technology
    Research Center

Chet de Groat
Professor of Pharmacology
University of Pittsburgh

John Donoghue
Director, Brain Science Program
Neuroscience Department
Brown University

Michael Dorman
Professor
Speech and Hearing Science
Arizona State University

Alexander Dromerick
Professor
Rehabilitation Medicine and
    Neurology Department
National Rehabilitation Hospital
Georgetown University

Donald Eigler
IBM Fellow
IBM Almaden Research Center

Jennifer Elisseeff
Assistant Professor
Biomedical Engineering
Johns Hopkins University

Leon Esterowitz
Program Director
Bioengineering and Environmental
    Systems
National Science Foundation

Boyd Evans
Research Staff
Biomedical Sciences
Oak Ridge National Laboratory

James Fallon
Professor
Anatomy and Neurobiology
University of California, Irvine

Gary K. Fedder
Howard M. Wilkoff Professor of
    ECE and Robotics
Director, Institute for Complex
    Engineered Systems
Carnegie Mellon University

Kirk Fernandes
Graduate Student/Journalist
Center for Science and Medical
    Journalism
Boston University

Harvey V. Fineberg
President
Institute of Medicine

Kate Fink
Graduate Student, Science
    Journalism
Boston University

Susan Fitzpatrick
Vice President
James S. McDonnell Foundation

Richard Foster
Managing Partner, Investment and
    Advisory Services LLC
Board Member, W. M. Keck
    Foundation

William Foster
Assistant Professor
Physics
The University of Houston

Joseph Francis
Assistant Professor
Department of Physiology and
    Pharmacology
State University of New York
    Downstate Medical Center

Robert C. Froemke
Postdoc
Department of Otolaryngology
University of California, San
    Francisco

Ken Fulton
Executive Director
National Academy of Sciences

Fred Gage
Vi and John Adler Professor
Laboratory of Genetics LOG-G
The Salk Institute of Biological
    Studies

Steven Gard
Research Associate Professor
Physical Medicine Rehabilitation
Northwestern University

Apostolos Georgopoulos
Regents Professor
Director, The Domenici Research
    Center for Mental Illness
    Department
University of Minnesota Medical
    School

Jeremy L. Gilbert
Professor and Associate Dean for
    Research
Biomedical and Chemical
    Engineering
Syracuse University

Brent Gillespie
Assistant Professor
Mechanical Engineering
University of Michigan

Simon Giszter
Associate Professor
Neurobiology and Anatomy
Drexel University College of
    Medicine

Steve Goldstein
Henry Ruppenthal Professor
Orthopaedic Surgery and
    Bioengineering Department
University of Michigan

Kevin Granata
Associate Professor
Musculoskeletal Biomechanics
    Laboratory
Virginia Tech

Elias Greenbaum
Corporate Fellow
Chemical Sciences Division
Oak Ridge National Laboratory

Warren M. Grill
Associate Professor
Biomedical Engineering and
    Surgery
Duke University

Selcuk Guceri
Dean
College of Engineering
Drexel University

Aparna Gupta
Assistant Professor
Decision Sciences and Engineering
    Systems
Rensselaer Polytechnic Institute

Brian Hafner
Research Director
Prosthetics Research Study

William Hammack
Professor
Chemical and Biomolecular
    Engineering
University of Illinois at Urbana-
    Champaign

Andrew Hansen
Research Assistant Professor
Physical Medicine and
    Rehabilitation
Northwestern University

Stuart Harshbarger
System Integrator
The Applied Physics Laboratory
Johns Hopkins University

Jiping He
Professor and Director
Bioengineering and Center for
    Neural Interface Design
Arizona State University

Anne Heberger
Research Associate
The National Academies
Keck Futures Initiative

William Heetderks
Director
Extramural Science Program
National Institute of Biomedical
    Imaging and Bioengineering
National Institutes of Health

Sarah Heilshorn
Assistant Professor
Materials Science and Engineering
Stanford University

Hugh Herr
Assistant Professor
Program in Media Arts and
    Sciences
Massachusetts Institute of
    Technology

Leigh Hochberg
Instructor / Investigator
Neurology / Neuroscience
    Department
Harvard Medical School /
Massachusetts General Hospital /
Brown University /
Veterans Administration Medical
    Center

Zhiyu ("Jerry") Hu
Research Scientist
Life Sciences Division
Oak Ridge National Lab

Gareth Hughes
Senior Engineer Biomedical
Zyvex Corporation

Mark Humayan
Professor of Ophthalmology
Associate Director of Research
Keck School of Medicine
Doheny Retina Institute
University of Southern California

Star Hy
Booz Allen Hamilton
SETA Support for Program
    Manager
DARPA/DSO

Pedro Irazoqui
Assistant Professor
Weldon School of Biomedical
 Engineering
Purdue University

Edwin Iversen
Vice President of Research and
 Development
Motion Control Inc.

Kenneth Jaffe
Professor, Rehabilitation Medicine
Adjunct Professor, Pediatrics and
 Neurological Surgery
Editor in Chief, Archives of
 Physical Medicine and
 Rehabilitation
University of Washington School
 of Medicine

Ranu Jung
Co-Director, Center for Adaptive
 Neural Systems, The
 Biodesign Institute
Associate Professor of
 Bioengineering
Arizona State University

Alla Katsnelson
Graduate Science Writing Student
University of California, Santa
 Cruz

Homayoon Kazerooni
Professor
Mechanical Engineering
University of California, Berkeley

Danielle Kerkovich, Ph.D.
Rehabilitation Research and
 Development Service
Department of Veterans Affairs

Robert Kirsch
Associate Professor of Biomedical
 Engineering
Case Western Reserve University

Zelma Kiss
Assistant Professor
Department of Clinical
 Neurosciences
University of Calgary

Elizabeth Kolbert
Staff Writer
The New Yorker

Jack Kotovsky
Engineer
Meso Micro and Nano Technology
Lawrence Livermore National
 Laboratory

Conrad Kufta
Director of Clinical Development
Innovative Neurotronics Inc.

Challa Kumar
Group Leader
Nanofabrication
Center for Advanced
 Microstructures and Devices
Louisiana State University

Themis Kyriakides
Assistant Professor
Biomedical Engineering and
    Pathology
Yale University

Joerg Lahann
Assistant Professor
Chemical Engineering and
    Biomedical Engineering
University of Michigan

Cato Laurencin
University Professor
Department of Orthopedic Surgery
University of Virginia Health
    System

Kendall Lee
Assistant Professor
Neurosurgery, Physiology,
    Biomedical Engineering, and
    Neurosurgery
Mayo Clinic Rochester

Irene W. Leigh, Ph.D.
Professor
Department of Psychology
Gallaudet University

Rachel Lesinski
Senior Program Specialist
The National Academies
Keck *Futures Initiative*

Hod Lipson
Assistant Professor
Mechanical and Aerospace
    Engineering
Cornell University

Treena Livingston Arinzeh
Assistant Professor
Biomedical Engineering
New Jersey Institute of Technology

Gerald Loeb
Professor, Biomedical Engineering
University of Southern California

Helen H. Lu
Assistant Professor, Biomedical
    Engineering
Columbia University

Charles C. Mann
Author

David Martin
Professor
Materials Science and Engineering
    Department
The University of Michigan

Yoky Matsuoka
Associate Professor
Computer Science and
    Engineering
University of Washington

Cameron McIntyre
Assistant Professor
Biomedical Engineering
Cleveland Clinic

Michael Merzenich
Francis Sooy Professor of
 Otolaryngology
Keck Center for Integrative
 Neurosciences
University of California, San
 Francisco, School of Medicine

Seth Messinger
Assistant Professor
Department of Sociology and
 Anthropology
University of Maryland, Baltimore
 County

Mahesh Mohanty
Project Manager
Advanced Technology
Stryker Orthopaedics

Pedram Mohseni
Assistant Professor
Electrical Engineering and
 Computer Science
Case Western Reserve University

David Mooney
Professor
Division of Engineering and
 Applied Sciences
Harvard University

Karen Moxon
Associate Professor
School of Biomedical Engineering
Drexel University

Naomi Murray
Senior Research Engineer
R&D—Technology Development
Stryker Orthopaedics

Vivian Mushahwar
Assistant Professor and AHFMR
 Scholar
Biomedical Engineering and
 Center for Neuroscience
University of Alberta

Isaac Mwase
Associate Professor of Philosophy
 and Bioethics
National Center for Bioethics,
 Tuskegee University

Hamid Najib
Personal Computer and Program
 Support Specialist
The National Academies

Erica Naone
Graduate Student
Science Writing
Massachusetts Institute of
 Technology

Roger Narayan
Associate Professor
Department of Biomedical
 Engineering
University of North Carolina

Richard Normann
Professor
Bioengineering Department
University of Utah

Randolph Nudo
Director, Landon Center on Aging
Professor, Molecular and
    Integrative Physiology
The University of Kansas Medical
    Center

Matthew O'Donnell
Dean
College of Engineering
University of Washington

Marcia O'Malley
Assistant Professor
Mechanical Engineering and
    Materials Science
Rice University

Santa Ono
Vice Provost and Deputy Provost
Emory University

Kevin Otto
Assistant Professor
Weldon School of Biomedical
    Engineering and Biological
    Sciences
Purdue University

Cengiz Ozkan
Assistant Professor
Mechanical Engineering
University of California, Riverside

Joseph Pancrazio
Program Director
Repair and Plasticity Cluster
    Department
Division Extramural Research
National Institute of Neurological
    Disorders and Stroke
National Institutes of Health

Hunter Peckham
Professor
Department of Biomedical
    Engineering
Case Western Reserve University

Maria Pellegrini
Vice President for Research
Brandeis University

Carlos Pena
Senior Science Policy Analyst
OC/OSHC
Food and Drug Administration

Marty Perreault
Program Director
The National Academies
Keck *Futures Initiative*

Haley Poland
Print Journalism Graduate Student
Annenberg School of
    Communication
University of Southern California

Alan Porter
Evaluation Coordinating
    Consultant
The National Academies
Keck *Futures Initiative*

Steve Potter
Assistant Professor
Laboratory for Neuroengineering
Georgia Institute of Technology

Elizabeth ("Beth") Quill
Graduate Science Writing Student
Massachusetts Institute of
    Technology

Sasha (Alexander) Rabchevsky
Assistant Professor of Physiology
Spinal Cord and Brain Injury
    Research Center
University of Kentucky

Walter Racette
Director
Certified Prosthetist/Orthotist
Assistant Clinical Professor
Department of Orthopaedic
    Surgery
University of California, San
    Francisco

Buddy Ratner
Professor
Bioengineering and Chemical
    Engineering
Director, University of Washington
    Engineered Biomaterials
    (UWEB)
University of Washington

Vilupanur Ravi
Professor
Chemical and Materials
    Engineering
California State Polytechnic
    University

Aristides Requicha
Gordon Marshall Chair in
    Engineering
Computer Science Department
University of Southern California

Frances Richmond
Director
Regulatory Science Program
School of Pharmacy
University of Southern California

Dave Roessner
Evaluation Consultant
The National Academies
Keck *Futures Initiative*

Robert Sah
Professor and Vice Chair
Department of Bioengineering
University of California, San Diego

Khaled Saleh
Associate Professor
Orthopedic Surgery
Division Head and Fellowship
    Director
Adult Reconstruction
University of Virginia

Gerwin Schalk
Research Scientist IV
Brain-Computer Interface R&D
    Program
Wadsworth Center, New York State
    Department of Health

Steven Schiff
Brush Chair Professor of
    Engineering
Center for Neural Engineering
The Pennsylvania State University

Elmar T. Schmeisser
Neurophysiology and Cognitive
    Neurosciences
U.S. Army Research Office

Karen Schrock
Science, Health, and
    Environmental Reporting
    Program
New York University

Joseph Schulman
President and Chief Scientist
Alfred Mann Foundation

Jeffrey Schwartz
Professor
Chemistry
Princeton University

Arthur M. Sherwood
Science and Technology Advisor
National Institute on Disability
    and Rehabilitation Research
Department of Education

Patricia Shewokis
Associate Professor and Movement
    Scientist
College of Nursing and Health
    Professions
Drexel University

Molly Shoichet
Professor and Director,
    Undergraduate Collaborative
    Bioengineering
Canada Research Chair in Tissue
    Engineering
University of Toronto

William Skane
Executive Director
Office of News and Public
    Information
The National Academies

Judith Stein
Chief Technologist
Chemical Nanotechnologies Lab
    Department
GE Global Research

Mercedes Talley
Program Director
W. M. Keck Foundation

Michael E. Tompkins
President
Animated Prosthetics Inc.

Dennis Turner
Professor
Neurosurgery, Neurobiology, and
    Neuroengineering
Duke University Medical Center

Dustin Tyler
Assistant Professor
Biomedical Engineering
Case Western Reserve University

Heinz Wässle
Professor, Doctor
Max-Planck-Institut

Michael Weinrich
Director
National Center for Medical
    Rehabilitation Research
National Institutes of Health

Bruce Wheeler
Professor and Interim Head
Bioengineering Department
University of Illinois

Blake Wilson
Senior Fellow
RTI International

George Wittenberg
Assistant Professor
Department of Neurology
University of Maryland
Geriatrics Research, Education,
    and Clinical Center
VA Maryland HCS

Wm. A. Wulf
President
National Academy of Engineering

Nic Young
Executive Producer
Lion House

Edyta Zielinska
Graduate Science Writing Student
New York University

Tom Zimmerman
Graduate Student
Grady College of Journalism and
    Mass Communication
The University of Georgia

Wendi Zongker
Graduate Student
Grady College of Journalism and
    Mass Communication
The University of Georgia